Yes I C

Researched, documented & proven protocols to disable, destroy and defeat cancer naturally.

by

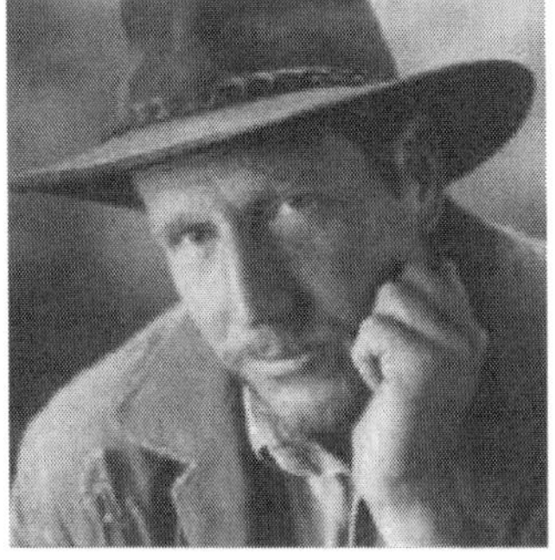

Michael Elliott

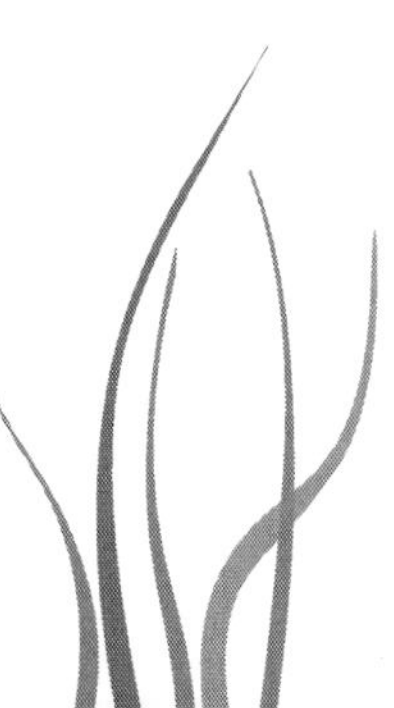

ISBN: 978-0-9897145-3-2

Disclaimer

The author of this book is not a doctor nor is he a physician. He has no medical license. Absolutely none of the information in this book is intended to be construed or used as medical advice. This book is the product of investigative journalism. That being said, the material in this book is for educational and informational purposes only. The choices and options for treatment are solely the decision of the individual. It is recommended that anyone with cancer or anyone that suspects he or she may have cancer, consult with a qualified physician.

A diligent and responsible effort has been made to provide accurate and authentic information. However the author cannot be held responsible for any inaccuracies that may be found in his source of materials and research. This also is not a comprehensive guide and or survey of all the non-toxic cancer treatments available, but rather treatments that the author feels are most important for the readers to know and learn about in their quest to regain their health.

Note: The Alternative Treatments and non-toxic protocols presented in this book are not approved by the FDA as treatments for cancer.

TABLE OF CONTENTS

Chapter 1

...What are my choices?...

"I look upon cancer in the same way that I look upon heart disease, arthritis, high blood pressure or even obesity, for that matter, in that by dramatically strengthening the body's immune system through diet, nutritional supplements, and exercise, the body can rid itself of the cancer, just as it does in other degenerative diseases. Consequently, I wouldn't have chemotherapy and radiation because I'm not interested in therapies that cripple the immune system, and, in my opinion, virtually ensure failure for the majority of cancer patients."

—Dr. Julian Whitaker, M.D.

"We have a multi-billion dollar industry that is killing people, right and left, just for financial gain. Their idea of research is to see whether two doses of this poison is better than three doses of that poison."

—Dr. Glen Warner, M.D. Oncologist.

If you are recently diagnosed with cancer and you are wondering if you should jump right into chemotherapy, radiation or surgery, you need to evaluate whether or not this is the wisest decision. Why would many physicians and oncologists refuse these treatments for their own family and friends?

Why would so many healthcare professionals refuse treatments that they commonly prescribe everyday to their own patients? Seems a bit odd don't you think? I think they know the damage these types of treatments can do to the human body and to the immune system. They know the statistics and they know the long term outcomes and survival rates from these common, overly prescribed protocols.

It's interesting to note how many doctors die of cancer. They seem to lose their battles at the same rate as the general public. I think far too many are totally ignorant or intentionally uninformed about alternative therapies. Another important conclusion would be, if doctors generally die at the same rate as the general public when diagnosed with cancer, why would you trust their advice when they can't even save themselves?.

Statistics reveal that nearly 75% of doctors and oncologists would refuse chemotherapy if diagnosed with cancer. Why? They see their patients and the effect chemotherapy has on their bodies. They watch the horrible suffering, the hair coming out in clumps, the weight loss, the nausea, the pain and the depression. Ironically, the percentage of patients with cancer that are prescribed chemotherapy, 75%.

The biggest factor of why they would refuse conventional therapies would have to be the statistics. They very cleverly manipulate the actual numbers, misleading the public into believing great strides have been made in cancer research and treatment. That we are ever so close to a cure. The brave researchers, scientists and doctors that have cured cancer ended up in prison, the morgue or disappeared into obscurity.

These doctors know that chemotherapy destroys and suppresses the immune system. Why on Earth would you give someone sick with cancer something that destroys the very thing that could possibly save them? How does this make any sense?.

Do we really see or hear about the actual, real life, personal experiences of patients that have decided to go the conventional route? Do we know what the majority of patients and family members go through mentally, physically, emotionally and financially when a loved one is diagnosed? What about the long and winding road ahead of them?

We see and hear advertisements about the state of the art, interactive treatment centers that work so hard to make that very personal and emotional connection. They seem to have a well rounded, caring and diverse group of professionals that assist and contribute to all aspects of the challenge ahead.

A challenge that will uncover who you really are. It will draw on the very strength and resoluteness of your character. The will and the fight that is within you. It is most definitely a journey. A journey into your Faith. Faith in your doctor, faith in your decisions, faith in God and faith in your resolve and courage to persist and prevail against all odds.

...Why should I listen to you? You're not a doctor...

That is true. I am not a doctor nor am I a physician. I have been extremely passionate about Natural/Holistic medicine for a little over 10 years and have a never ending drive for more and more understanding and knowledge. The information in this book is as accurate as possible and will hopefully help as a guide you can use to weigh out your options and alternative possibilities.

I will attempt to give you a brief example of my journey as the caregiver and spouse of a cancer alumni. Of course her journey differed greatly from mine on many levels but we were bonded and devoted by the virtue of our vows, before God, to travel this road together.

The research and information confirming the efficacy and successes of alternative medicine is overwhelming. It needs to be available as an option in your upcoming battle. Everyone should have the choice to decide for themselves what they are willing to subject their bodies too, conventional or natural.

I am an Herbalist and have been studying Naturopathic and Holistic medicine for a little over 10 years. I am also an Artist, Craftsman, and was an active Nevada State Firefighter before this life changing cancer diagnosis.

I am extremely fond of books and have a never ending desire and intensity to learn. I have a very good understanding of first aid and how to deal with major trauma being a first responder for the fire department. Other than that, I was totally new to the concept of cancer and how it came to afflict so many. Searching for the truth and finding logical answers is my passion.

...How did this happen...

The problem is that once the body falls victim to an affliction such as cancer, the whole body is involved in the process of disease. Sure, the cancer may have set up shop in one specific area of the body, typically the weakest link or organ but, for this issue to have manifested and formed, something went terribly wrong with your body's innate ability to recognize and destroy this foreign invader. The immune system was not firing on all cylinders.

It only stands to reason that the environment and workings of the entire or whole body need to be addressed. How can you possibly focus on one specific area of the body and expect a lifelong or enduring recovery? How can you guarantee or at least offer the hope that it will not return without addressing the reason behind the breakdown in the first place.

Everything in our body is tied together, it all works in a systematic, synergistic conglomeration. When we have a breakdown or failure of a specific part, we create an imbalance in the body. The body, being as smart as it is, will do its best to try and work around or find an alternative to the malfunctioning part.

This malfunctioning part will affect another area being that everything relies on everything else to do its job. It creates a type of snowball effect that eventually leads to disease or dis-ease within our body chemistry.

Conventional medicine will either remove the affected area or mass, if possible, surgically, offer up targeted radiation treatment or they will advise whole body poisoning with chemotherapy. There are definitely times and places for conventional medicine. It is not always, as most typically assume, your best and most reliable choice. Whatever direction you choose to pursue, you have to decide if this is the course of action you can live with, literally, live with.

I know that healthcare professionals and doctors do not intentionally want to harm their patients, even though, prescribing these toxic cocktails and treatments can inflict irreparable damage to the body and its organs.

A large percentage of healthcare professionals have never been educated or trained in the art of enabling the body to work it's own miracles. They would rather induce their own, man-made, so called "miracles". They know they are not addressing the underlying cause and the ultimate initiation of the disease. They also know it could return at anytime.

They are left in a kind of "keep your fingers crossed" mentality. That doesn't really work for me. I don't know about you, but it would be nice to have something a little bit more substantial. I was never one to rely too much on luck, and to trust your life to a roll of the dice is madness. Also, their real life, realistic survival statistics are dismal at best.

If you are comfortable with that picture and potential outcome and you think you can be faithful and diligent in your daily prayers, than that is what most people will decide to do. It will take a large support group of people praying for you daily no matter which course of treatment you decide upon. There is energy and power in prayer.

If by chance you believe and understand that your internal and external environment are responsible for this cancer and or disease, and that your body is capable of repairing the damage by changing that environment, then you should, by all accounts, continue investigating your alternatives and options. At least make your decision from a better understanding of how and why these alternatives work.

...Personal Story...

I have firsthand experience with cancer and its typical applications and treatments. My wife was diagnosed with stage IV non-small cell, adenocarcinoma of the lung at the age of 41.

She did not smoke although non-small cell is typically not associated with smoking. She did suffer from a lifelong asthma condition. She was on the typically prescribed albuterol inhaler a few times a day for tens of years, ever since she was a child. Did the albuterol after so many years initiate her lung cancer? Nobody knows, your guess is as good as mine.

Albuterol is a totally foreign, chemical mist you inhale into your lungs as needed. Anytime she had any kind of gasps for air or shortness of breath she would engage her inhaler. Maybe the potential for cancer is listed in the small book of side effects. I'm sure the manufacturer's covered their bases just in case it caused some dreadful disease down the road.

There are far too many pharmaceutical drugs prescribed that they have no idea what potential long term manifestations might appear. So, they have page after page of disclaimers right? But who reads those crazy things anyways.

We would never take any of the prescribed medications if we really tried to digest all the potential side effects from taking the drug. And that's no fun! Were all about fast and easy, no work, give me the pill anyways, right? I don't want to have to work for my health or deny myself whatever I want, give me the magic cap and make me all better. God we're lazy.

It was a total surprise diagnosis. The doctor thought she probably pulled a muscle riding her horse and suggested she should take it easy for a couple of weeks until the sharp pain in her chest subsided a bit. We tried that but about a week later she sat up in bed in extreme pain. The sharp, stabbing pain was not getting better so, at 2 am in the morning we rushed to emergency.

They calmed her down with a sedative or two and decided on an x-ray to be sure. Voila, there it was, they diagnosed her with pneumonia and sent her home with some heavy duty antibiotics and pain medication. We were really hoping that the pain medication and the antibiotics would kick in within a few days but, unfortunately, she shot up in bed again a few nights later.

We went back to the doctor. This time we were sent to a respiratory specialist and he claimed that 1 out of a 100 patients had issues resolving the infection on the first go round so, he recommended another round of antibiotics and tried to send us home again.

I tried to explain to him that being that 1 in a 100 wasn't working for me and pleaded for further testing to nail down the diagnosis of pneumonia. I knew how serious pneumonia could get and I didn't want to take any chances.

He argued that the only other possible test would be a needle biopsy and that it was too dangerous, he might puncture a lung. We went back and forth for what seemed like an exaggerated length of time until he finally relented and decided to keep her overnight for the biopsy.

Unfortunately the pain increased substantially that night and they administered morphine to reduce the discomfort and pain. She had a major reaction to the morphine and her heart rate skyrocketed. She nearly died from this questionable event.

Early the next morning they performed the needle biopsy of her lung. Everything seemed to have gone well with the procedure thankfully, so now all we had to do was wait. Waiting can make you crazy when your dealing with frightening potentials. We got a call the next day from the receptionist at her respiratory physicians office and were told we had an appointment right away to see the doctor.

We thought the worst and assumed the pneumonia was extremely serious and had gotten worse. Damn, I knew it. Why else would a doctors office accommodate us so quickly and efficiently, definitely not their M.O.

When we arrived at his office they led us in right away. The doctor was rather solemn and proceeded to inform us that we had an appointment with the oncologist next door. The biopsy had confirmed positive results for cancer.

We walked in complete shock to the oncologists office questioning how this could be, she didn't smoke, she always made sure she ate a decent square meal and filled up a couple of bottles of good quality water every morning. She was supposed to be the healthy one.

Thinking back, she said her asthma symptoms had changed recently, her cough was different and something was just a little off. I tried for 6 months to get her to go see the doc but she stubbornly refused over and over.

I finally made an appointment for her and told her that she had to go. She refused again. So much for my authority and her respecting that authority. I'm sure you all know what I'm talking about. It's called the severely stubborn spouse syndrome.

If you are faced with anything questionable medically, do whatever you have to do to get them to go. Do not pass it off as I did and relented to her just being stubborn. I tried everything I could think of to get her to go but for naught. I even threatened to take her precious ice cream away. Even that failed! She is very strong willed and oh did I mention, stubborn!

Well, a month later I made another appointment for her and she adamantly refused for the 3rd or 4th time, I can't remember, I've lost track of her insubordination. Really pushes my limits when I think of how much less advanced her cancer may have been had she decided to do the safe thing and at least get things checked out a long time ago.

So, we are quietly waiting for our face to face with the oncologist, everything is surreal. This isn't really happening right? I mean she looks fine and feels fine except for this sharp shooting type pain in her chest. This is a cancer doctor, these people look really sick, they are all wearing beanies or fancy scarves, their knocking on deaths door. These people are dying!

We are eventually invited in to his office and seated. The anticipation of his words was psychologically debilitating. I can't think straight, Janie seems scared but hopeful, she always is.

...The Diagnosis...

The doctor re-examines and shuffles through the films in front of him, looks over at our dismay and dis-belief and says "I'm very sorry but this does not look hopeful." He politely tells us that his diagnosis would be stage IV lung cancer. He sees the anguish in our faces and then tells us that there is probably not much he can do at this point. He estimates 6-9 months at best.

"Excuse me I say, do you mean that she only has 6-9 months left to live and that there is virtually nothing you can do to change that?" Not a sliver of hope, not even the possibility for a turn of the cards? He tells us we can try some chemotherapy but without much hope of effect. He suggests a second opinion through the UC Davis oncology department in Sacramento.

We decided that this Carson City, Nevada oncologist was badly mistaken and that a second opinion from such a reputable, well known institute like UC Davis would be wise. So we made our appointment for as soon as possible. The clock was ticking away the minutes, hours and days, how many did she have left? They seemed to be flying by so fast except when we were waiting for results or further testing.

We had our meeting with the oncologist at UC Davis and he suggested the possibility that the cancer could be resected. He said he would discuss her situation and options in their group meeting of physicians the next day.

He was very optimistic so we were finally very excited that something could be done. I'm of course thinking, oh my God, is this oncologist in Carson City a complete idiot? Is there a reason his name is Dr. Bleak?

Why and how do you completely wipe out anyone's chance for hope. There is always hope, if you have Faith, you have hope, it is always there. Faith, Hope and Love. The big 3, right? We had the love and we always had the Faith. The 3 have to go together if you want to survive.

This doctor at UC Davis even proposed a possible complete resection and removal of the cancer. Wow, what an amazing sense of relief! We scheduled a return visit a couple of days later and anxiously awaited our new found optimism in at least having the potential for choices, choices for life and for defeating this ugly beast.

Of course we were early for our appointment, I think I just paced for two whole days pondering the possibilities of such a huge, life changing decision. Holy crap, if we, or I, made the wrong decision, how could I live with myself if it turned out to be the wrong one.

What a horrible predicament people have to face when confronted with this dilemma of choice, this crucial, there's no room for a mistake decision. Of course we are being led by the conventional way of attack and logic. This is their business, their livelihood, they certainly are not going to recommend the local Healer or Shaman as an option.

Way too many thoughts go through your mind and it's very difficult to turn it off. A constant rerun of potential outcomes. In the end I had to learn to give it to God or succumb to my own form of insanity. Somehow God would guide my steps if only I could just be still.

On our return visit to UC Davis we didn't actually get to see the original doctor as he was busy in surgery, so, another doctor filled in. I think he may have been embarrassed about his overly enthusiastic expression of hopefulness. I really don't think he was in surgery. I think that was proof of how much they truly care, he couldn't face the devastating news we were about to receive, at least that's what I felt in my gut.

Maybe he really was in surgery or maybe he was just overly saddened by his offer of hope being taken apart by his colleagues. I know they genuinely want to help their patients. They want to save your life, that's what they signed up for.

Anyways, the stand in doctor stated that Dr. Oops was sadly mistaken about the potential to remove the cancer, and that our only option was IV chemotherapy, and with that only a slight chance of any success or the possibility of remission. Sooooo, back to Carson City and Dr. Bleak.

At this point Dr. Bleak tells us that he can help manage her pain and keep her comfortable. We are still in denial and total shock. She was chucking hay to the horses last night and now she is going to be dead in 6-9 months. Great! This has to be a mistake.

This couldn't and shouldn't have happened to her. So began my frantic study and education of alternative cancer treatments and therapies.

It was really frustrating trying to understand why Janie would not agree to certain protocols. Some of them were really simple too. One of the protocols was the Flaxseed Oil and Cottage Cheese Protocol. I mentioned before that she was very stubborn and she was very adamant and resolved that this was not going to be a protocol she would submit to.

It was strange I guess that she relied on me more than the doctors on advising her on what she should be doing. We really didn't know where else to go. She complied with just about all of my investigative research. I was at a loss why she so strongly refused methods and modalities that I had great hope for. I know there are many I will never quite understand.

She would not even give this Flaxseed Oil and Cottage Cheese protocol a chance. She just turned her nose up at it. She would also not go along with the Gerson Therapy. I had great hope for this method of treatment also but, she would only drink maybe 1 or 2 smoothies a day and they had to be really flavorful. There was no way she would attempt the 13 glasses of juice required on the Gerson Therapy. It was excruciatingly frustrating. She did do pretty well with a multitude of daily supplements, I just had to sit there and coax her to take them all.

I started out with her taking Beta Glucans, Juice Plus (a whole food supplement containing 17 fruits and vegetables), IP6, Maitake and Shiitake mushrooms, Olive Leaf Extract, Spirulina, Red Clover tops tea (3-4 times a day), Pau D' Arco, B17 (Laetrile, 500mg tablets), Milk Thistle, MGN-3 (although during the course of her treatment the FDA removed this super cancer killing supplement from the health food store shelves), Ellagic acid, Poly MVA, Essiac Tea, Grapeseed extract, Vitamin C and others.

Of course I didn't have her on all of these at the same time. I would try a few, find out about another 1 or 2, change ones I thought might be better and so forth. I had to take into consideration that I could only get her to take so many at a time and so many in a day. It was quite the challenge. Deciding which to take and which not to take, which were too expensive for everyday and God help me so many other variables I lost track.

If only I had this book back then. Don't get me wrong, there were stacks of amazing books I was referring to and I'm really grateful to the outstanding and courageous authors, I know the research and love they put into their work.

Part of it was just not knowing anything about any of this. At the same time I was trying to make sense out of information overload. Trying to absorb so much information so fast and then trying to decide which therapy had the greatest potential was draining. I was doing my best to try and figure out what was worth pursuing and what we might be able to afford. I was her backyard, constantly evolving, alternative, redneck doctor. When I hit a block wall with her refusals to try a new therapy it was mass panic and confusion all over again, I had spent too much time investigating this next wave of attack.

I did get her to drink 2-3 glasses of mostly carrot juice along with an apple and a stalk or 2 of celery added in. These were daily as long as I could get her to drink it. She was really up for just about whatever the first couple of years. She was mostly a good sport. It was her dismissing alternative treatments that had a proven track record that flustered me.

I did end up purchasing the organic ingredients to brew the Essiac Tea myself at home. That one was easy to administer. It was 3 ounces, 3 times a day on an empty stomach. I made sure I purchased the Essiac Tea that included the roots of the Sheep Sorrel herb. That was a mandatory requirement for the real formula. There are a lot of varieties out there but, the original recipe was the 4 herbs. Burdock Root, Sheep Sorrel, Turkey Rhubarb and Slippery Elm Bark.

After sorting things out a bit more and trying to determine what we could afford, I tried to make sure she took 6-8,000mg of Vitamin C daily, MGN3 (while it was available), Beta-Glucans (Maitake D-fraction), Juice Plus (17 fruits & vegetables in a capsule), Noni juice, 1-2 lemons a day in a little bit of warm water and 2-3 additional smoothies a day when I could. The smoothies got really expensive too and we were nowhere near being well off financially.

I used watermelon, red beets, blueberries, wheatgrass, alfalfa sprouts, a plain live culture yogurt and a banana (I tried different combinations with broccoli and asparagus too, I just had to add certain things to make her want to drink it, otherwise she would just hand it back to me and tell me to drink it. I also had her take a balanced, ionic mineral supplement and Amygdalin 500mg (Laetrile). Unfortunately we could not afford to keep up with many of these supplements and juice drinks.

I think that is one of the greatest personal defeats. When you have so much faith in a particular supplement or treatment and the person's life hangs in the balance but you can't afford it. A big slap for me. Makes you feel less than adequate when you can't afford to potentially save your spouse's life. I spent our house and my business, I didn't have anything left to spend.

We did get help here and there. We had an amazing country community that held a very well attended fundraiser. The entire town was involved and many people went way out of their way to make it a huge success. One of the main organizers of the fundraiser was another amazing friend, one of those people that seemed happy all the time and was always helping somebody out. He was fine at the time of the fundraiser but would end up losing his life to colon cancer before Janie.

My brother and his wife's family were always ready to help wherever and whenever they could. Our church even donated money. A very good friend at the local flower shop donated a huge amount of time and effort organizing many things. Besides everything else they did, our friends down the street, towards the end, would come down and help bathe Janie, get her into to some clean clothes and change her bed sheets. The friends we got together with nearly every weekend, whether she felt horrible or not, would drop everything at a moments notice. Everyone went out of their way to do what they could to give me a break.

My beautiful sister stayed with me the last week or two, 24/7. It would have been so much harder without her presence. Janie even had a close horseback riding friend from Wyoming buy a trailer and move onto the property to help take care of her.

I had a local woman volunteer to do our books and our taxes. She was extraordinarily generous with her time and talents. She stuck close to me even after Janie passed helping with anything and everything, including helping me pack up the place after I unsuccessfully failed to save the house. The spoils of war. I lost all the way around. I owe this kind woman so much, and someday I will return the blessing that she has been to me. These were all down home, country loving type of folks. They seemed to join forces when someone in the valley was in need. I am so grateful and will never forget what everyone did for us!

Sometimes humanity shines. Sometimes, something takes precedence over our daily affray. Sometimes the noise and the clutter of life simply fades and the love of the heart overwhelms and permeates the void.

So many busy people in a very chaotic life found the time to offer up what they could. In the meantime, life changing events were in constant motion. Life events really change your focus and place your attention on the simple beauty of the moment. We spend so much time lost in the past and thoughts of the future, we forget to enjoy the right now. It seems we blink our eyes and our world changes. It happened to my closest childhood friend. The ironies of life.

My best friend Jake that I grew up with lived about an hour north in Lake Tahoe. His wife used to call Janie almost daily just to keep her spirits going. Of course it didn't take much. If you heard her on the phone, which was several times a day, (she had way too many friends), you would never even know she was sick. She would be laughing and joking, comforting somebody else and offering advice to their problems. She was not one to remain seated on the self-pity pot! I really couldn't help but admire her state of mind. I think she just had that much faith in God and He was definitely testing her faith.

At least that's what she thought, I think it at least kept her motivated to persevere. I remember one of her favorite Bible verses was Psalm 118:17-21. "I will not die; instead, I will live to tell what the Lord has done. The Lord has punished me severely, but He did not let me die. Open for me the gates where the righteous enter, and I will go in and thank the Lord. These gates lead to the presence of the Lord, and the Godly enter there. I thank you for answering my prayer and giving me victory!"

Anyway, back to the story. My best friend Jake and his wife had also been together a long time. Jake came back from dirt bike riding one weekend and found his wife a little under the weather, actually a little more than under the weather. Her skin was sallow, somewhat yellow and her energy level was waning. He pleaded with her to go to the hospital but had no luck. Seems there are a lot of stubborn women out there. It was nice to know others had the same problem as me.

After 2-3 weeks of getting progressively worse, she finally relented and agreed to go to the hospital. It's a long story, complete with a gross misdiagnosis from her doctors at the hospital. The wrong treatment, the wrong drugs and the wrong assumptions. This mistake would end up taking her life about a year before Janie passed. My closer than a brother BFF was devastated, a sad and excruciating painful taste of unexpected shock and life altering grief.

This life can really throw you a fast ball to the gut sometimes. We lost another good friend during all this in a rain soaked mudslide in central California. All of these close friends that passed were somewhere in their forties, they were all young guns. It's just the irony of Janie being given a death sentence from her doctors, (6-9 months) and then so many close friends, young close friends, moving on to the Father ahead of her, strange days indeed. I know it was Janie's attitude and her diet that was extending her life.

So, besides the supplements she tried her best to take daily, I made alkaline water for her to drink. I put 2 pouches of an Okinawan Coral Calcium in her purified water. The raw coral calcium in the packets slowly leaches into the water. I also put 8-10 drops of "Cell Food" (this comes in a small bottle at the health food store). She pretty much had the water with her constantly. I basically relied on her diet, the smoothies and the liquid supplements to get the recommended vitamins. The Juice Plus too. From my exhausting research I just don't believe in isolated or multivitamins. I have more confidence in God's packaging, not man's. No offense "man."

Another therapy we tried was the Hoxsey Therapy. We went to Mexico to the clinic and purchased the formula. We continued on the formula for around 3 months and then ran out of money again. It's really hard to determine whether or not anything was working except monitoring how she was feeling. But then again, that was not a very accurate assessment. She was feeling fine when she was diagnosed with stage IV lung cancer.

Of course, since we were now in alternative treatment land, we couldn't just order up some conventional tests to see how she was progressing. Insurance didn't cover anything obscure or as bizarre as building the immune system. It had to be surgery, radiation or chemo, no exceptions.

The oncologist that was managing her cancer and pain medications eventually ordered up some new scans. He wanted to see how much further her cancer had progressed. He was also a bit curious as to how she was still alive. When he got the scans back he scheduled us for an office visit. He told us that he had some good news.

Apparently, nearly all of the cancer in her lungs had mysteriously disappeared. It was too difficult to distinguish between the lung cancer and scar tissue. I don't think I will ever forget the look on his face. I think Janie and I both blacked out for a moment. Then I said, What? You mean the death sentence you originally gave us with no hope for a recovery is null and void? He replied, "Yes, from what I see on the scans, that seems to be the case." This was the miracle we had been praying for. This nearly always fatal stage IV lung cancer was in severe remission. The cancer was seemingly being destroyed by Janie's supercharged immune system.

The doctor was also a bit curious as to what we were doing. He told us to continue with whatever we were doing and that he would monitor her progress with another set of scans in a few months.

We continued with the therapies as best we could and as best we could afford. Something was working. Which one I could only pray would be one of the ones I chose to keep her on daily, whether we were in the middle of a broke phase again or not. What a crazy ride, you can't buy a ticket for one of these. The experience is free, the decisions you have to make are expensive and they can cost you your life.

So, what really healed the lung cancer? I don't know. I'm thinking it was a little bit of everything. Everything I just mentioned. It truly is a whole new world trying to treat someone medically with alternatives instead of mainstream, political medicine.

We were doing all the right things, or so it seemed. Looking back, I still think the biggest issue was not doing a thorough enough job of cleansing her intestinal tract and her colon. If only we had implemented the coffee enemas and stayed with it. If only we had been able to continue with the Hoxsey Therapy, the Laetrile (Amygdalin), the Essiac Tea, the Noni Juice and the other somewhat expensive supplements, then what? They go fast when you are taking 2-6 of them a day.

...Connected to the Earth...

I also made sure she spent some time out in the Sun for 20-30 minutes everyday. Just not during peak hours and certainly not with any sunscreen. I now know that spending some time out in the Sun with your bare feet connected to the Earth is very stimulating and healing. The Earth is our greatest antioxidant. Connecting to it daily with your bare feet should be a mandatory part of any recovery. Believe it or not the Earth's electrical surface charge is always abundantly filled with negatively charged, free electrons.

Electrons are the smallest negative charge of electricity. Negatively charged free electrons have an affinity for positive charged free radicals. That just means they like them. This inhibits free radicals from oxidizing healthy tissue. This in turn, reduces chronic inflammation and pain associated with degenerative disease.

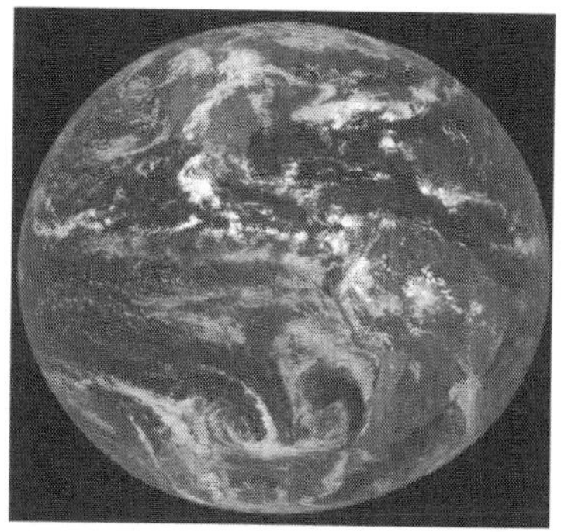

Tests conducted with infrared thermal imaging after being grounded to the Earth was dramatic. This thermal imaging analyzes the skins surface temperature, differentiating between normal and inflamed areas of the body. Thermal imaging is used to diagnose many common physiological disorders. Diabetes, breast cancer, nervous system abnormalities, headaches, chronic and acute pain, sprains, arthritis, carpal tunnel syndrome, arterial disease and more.

Patients involved in the study were grounded to the Earth through grounded conductive electrodes or grounded bed pads. Some patients reported positive results after just one session. Others, with ongoing ½ hour treatments 2 or 3 times a week, reported noticeable relief and that they felt better overall. Others after several weeks and months reported their symptoms had disappeared altogether.

The thermal images of patients before and after being grounded for as little as 30 minutes, another being grounded for 4 nights on a grounded bed pad are impressive. The visible reduction in heat and inflammation on the images is inspiring. I'm sure not everyone will experience these same type of results as there are other factors determining the outcome.

Regardless, grounding, in my opinion, is just another one of God's grand designs we know nothing about. I just think that everything we need to heal is right in front of us and it's free. The Sun, the water, the Earth, the air, the plants, the trees, etc. Kick your shoes off, go for a walk, feel the Earth move under your feet.

Being grounded to the Earth also improved their sleep patterns and reduced and normalized their levels of cortisol, our stress induced hormone. Without starting a completely new chapter, I kind of did but I just wanted to put some information in here without getting into too much detail. Get out in the Sun, go for a walk in your bare feet, absorb the natural healing energies from the Earth, it's free and it really isn't going to hurt you. You need to get out of the house anyways. Okay now, where was I? Oh yeah.

Janie was the kind of person who ended up being your best friend after meeting her for the first time. You know those people who make you crazy because they are rarely sad and are always ready to share a smile and always looking for a reason to laugh. That was Janie, that was just the way she was wired. Her mother was an equally amazing lady and a great help to us always. I couldn't have custom ordered a better second mother. You didn't dare succumb to the self-pity pot when she was around, that just wasn't a behavior she tolerated or believed in. Her favorite word for a long time was "Happiness" This wasn't one of those times.

The support from family and friends was a blessing. Her cousin and his wife would travel a very long distance just to make food for us. Her brothers and our nieces and nephews were also extremely helpful and kept in contact with Janie.

Our best friends were local Deputy Sheriffs. We spent at least every weekend eating Roseannes amazing cooking and playing some silly board game. They also went above and beyond with anything we needed. Roseanne and Janie used to ride horseback together just about every week. I really do miss them all! Janie just had a huge support network. All of this love reflected on the kind of person she was.

I'm sure her personality was the reason why the memorial service was standing room only. I think about that sometimes, what are you like? How many people do you think will show up to your memorial service? Sad that we never find out what people really thought of us until after we're gone. The attendance at your memorial service says a lot about the type of person you were. Don't be afraid to let your light shine, make sure the world knows who the real you is, Janie did, make sure you fill the church too.

By the way she made it nearly 4 years. She passed on to the next world and into the ever loving arms of our Creator God the Father, February 9, 2007. The alternative treatments were working, but which one or ones? Like I said before, I'm really not sure to be perfectly honest. She made it way past the original 6-9 month diagnosis. My problem was I had my hand in too many baskets, which basket held the key? That's the saddest part. Then this brain metastasis thing pops up out of nowhere. Now what?

The stage IV lung cancer had virtually disappeared and reduced to scar tissue. We thought we had defeated the beast. We thought we were going to be the face of God's grace and hope for cancer patients everywhere. We had really big plans. I guess that was all just an illusion.

Nearly 2 ½ years after the initial lung cancer diagnosis she started having headaches. I figured it was from the severely damaging chemotherapy treatments we attempted. The chemicals were trying to find their way out of her body. At least that's what we were hoping.

Unfortunately the headaches were not the toxins trying to clear her system. Turns out the cancer had metastasized to her brain. That one came straight out of a Rocky Horror Picture Show. More shock, more disbelief, more confusion, more education and more late nights studying. Studying till I literally fell asleep on a book or on the computer keyboard.

Eventually we figured this metastasized brain cancer was just another bump in the road she had to overcome or we had to overcome, we were in this together. I ended up having to turn away clients for my business simply because she needed full time care. It was that "in sickness and in health" promise we both made to God.

I had been studying how difficult it was to cross that blood brain barrier with any kind of treatment. Why was this seemingly starting all over again. We had seemingly defeated the lung cancer and now, a new dance we knew nothing about. This was a completely different world, especially dealing with the confined spaces of the skull. So naturally we panicked again and followed the educated advice of the oncologist who recommended setting her up for radiation treatments right away. We didn't even have time to think it over.

It wasn't until later, after the radiation treatments were completed that I found out that they typically only extend the life of the patient a month or two. Besides that, the radiation treatment itself causes cancer. This is getting way too confusing, why would they prescribe something so foreboding and malicious. I couldn't get the why's out of my head.

Her immune system was so strong at this point she struggled with the brain cancer for nearly a year and a half. Thing I didn't realize through all my research was that her system needed to be more thoroughly cleaned out, her organs of elimination needed a precise and over the top cleansing and a strict, no cheating, alkaline, cancer diet.

It's really hard to determine what is effective and what is not when you choose to do a detox. What this needed to involve was certainly not your basic detox. Something had gone dreadfully wrong with her immune system for this to have manifested in the first place. Would supplements be strong enough? Would they really do the trick? Were they reliable? What do I look for and how do I know if they are powerful enough to do what needed to be done?

I think I just sort of skimmed past the coffee enema thing. Being green, I guess it just sounded too ridiculous to be of any benefit. Now, looking back at where I was and where I am now, the coffee enema is one of the first things I would do, damn! Hindsight is a horrible thing to try and live with. It was one of those wrong decision things I was so worried about.

Where and what do you start with first? Sure, I read ad after ad and page after page of supplements for liver cleanse, kidney flush, bowel care etc. Was that really all there was to it? Just pop a bottle or two of some miraculous supplements and that would do the trick? It really is a rough road trying to decipher what's legit, what's marketing, and what has to happen in what order.

Although her immune system was really strong we were more or less pouring good clean virgin oil on top of a very dirty engine. Most people and most supplements do a very gentle, skim the surface type of cleansing. We needed to get to the caked on sludge at the bottom of the barrel. You know, the stuff that won't come off no matter what you try.

We needed to get out the hammer and a cold chisel. We and or she had been eating chemically laced, processed, adulterated foods for a very long time. Skimming the surface with a gentle, comfortable, nearly void of any side effects detox was blatantly inadequate.

Naturally we did everything we could think of to try and fend off the new dilemma of conquering this brain cancer, after all, we were going to be the face of hope and perseverance for cancer patients everywhere. We even traveled to the renowned Burzynski cancer clinic in Houston, Texas. We had mixed results there, although the tumors had responded somewhat. The doctor at the Burzynski clinic told us that their treatment would be limited in its effect simply because she had already been through radiation treatments.

We were determined to stay away from any further conventional treatments. Their outlook and recommendations were rather pessimistic anyways. Plus she didn't want to have to deal with the side effects all over again.

Fortunately, the doctor was only prescribing whatever pain meds he thought would keep her comfortable. The initial IV chemotherapy failures, sadly, did not have any effect except for the misery of the side effects with her hair falling out in clumps, the nausea, diarrhea, headaches, fatigue and sleeplessness. We were pretty much on our own after the initial 3-4 months.

In the beginning when he did attempt the chemotherapy, we pretty much knew he was only doing it to appease us and attempt something. He told us there was not much hope for success. It's kind of like the fire department showing up for a fire that is fully involved. We put water on the fire partly for show. We pretty much know there isn't a chance of saving the structure but, to keep up appearances and to do our job, we needed to squirt some water. So that's what the oncologist did, squirt some water. He just replaced the water with poison, I mean chemo.

I was constantly, and to this day, wondering how much more intense and powerful her immune system might have been had we not relented to the chemotherapy. The chemotherapy does untold damage to the immune system and organs. What if we had decided to go all natural treatments? I knew the "what if's" would create problems and leave far too many unanswered questions down the road. Eventually I had to let them go.

I kept analyzing the questions of how this brain metastasis manifested in the first place. If her immune system was strong enough to eradicate and decimate the lung cancer, how did it come to rear its ugly head in her brain? I keep going back to the colon cleansing.

The lung cancer was obviously well developed and advanced at stage IV. With her immune system so powerful and strong, maybe all the dead and dying toxic cancer cells from the lung never completely made their way out of her system. Maybe because we didn't do a thorough enough job of clearing up her systemic constipation.

With her inefficient bowel movements, maybe the leftover toxins from the lung cancer re-circulated back into her bloodstream and body fluids. Maybe she would have been fine if her organs of elimination and colon had been completely cleared and performing perfectly. Maybe because we never addressed and flushed out the caked on sludge in her colon, her body couldn't handle the extra burden. Maybe it was all about her body not being able to effectively eliminate this toxic debris fast enough. I think this was my most painful mistake and the primary reason behind the metastasis.

I guess that is part of the reason I repeat myself so many times in this book. When you start killing off the cancer, it has to have an exit. A clearly defined and labeled evacuation route. No limits, no boundaries, no back up, no waiting, here's the door! Get out, your not welcome here anymore! Please do not overlook this, I know I will keep reminding you.

We did finally make an appointment with a Homeopath/Oncologist in Reno. We had heard good things about him and decided to give him a try.

He put her on IV Vitamin C and Laetrile (Vitamin B17) once a week. That was actually showing some really great progress so we continued with that along with all the supplements and other protocols we were able to afford.

The scans were showing improvement and that the tumors were shrinking. We were really excited that the intravenous vitamin C and B17 (laetrile) was having such an impact. The longer we continued with this therapy the more promising the possibility for a complete reversal of this newest nightmare. We finally had something positive to be excited about, again.

After about 3-4 months of promising results on this therapy we went in for our weekly procedure and treatment when the doctor took us aside. He informed us that the FDA had pretty much overnight, made it illegal to administer B17 (Laetrile) anymore and that his hands were completely tied. They threatened to take away his medical license if he continued.

Apparently the Laetrile was having extremely positive results at several different alternative cancer clinics and the pharmaceutical powerhouse decided to flex their influence with the FDA and have it removed through some legalistic loopholes. They succeeded and it is no longer legal to use it as a treatment here in the U.S.

We did continue with the IV vitamin C therapy once a week. I wish the doctor had emphasized the importance of continuing with a thorough detox regimen. A regimen that would dive deeper into her systemic constipation dilemma. He was still managing her discomforts with pain medication, anxiety medication and something to help her sleep which only compounded the problem.

She was definitely not having regular enough bowel movements, and when she did, it was nothing worthy of headlines. Nobody ever mentioned the dire necessity and effectiveness of coffee enema's or seeing a colon hydro-therapist. Something or anything that would help relieve her body of these dead and dying, toxic cancer cells. Something that would help facilitate the release and removal of all the accumulated and impacted fecal debris.

I now completely believe that this impacted fecal debris from a lifetime of tainted foods not only kept her from eliminating the dying cancer cells from the lung but severely limited the amount of available and absorb-able nutrients from all the powerful supplements and cancer fighting, alkaline foods she was taking.

I guess I was expecting more from this Homeopath/Oncologist. I was hoping that he would be our savior and that I could take some sort of break from the constant need for more information. If he didn't bring it up then I just assumed that what we or I were doing was sufficient. That all our ducks were lining up. It obviously was not what I had hoped.

He was a very caring and heart of the matter physician. He had so many patients he was trying to help. I'm not blaming him at all. He would even personally call to see how Janie was doing after his practice closed for the day. You could tell he was crushed when they took away the Laetrile.

After awhile the tumors started growing again. Possibly from the removal of the Laetrile. The vitamin C and the Laetrile needed each other. They were very effective when utilized in combination with one another. So sad, such needless and avoidable suffering. I'm not even going to ask why. I know why. Here was a natural substance that was effective, it was helping, it was healing. It may have changed her fate.

So many days so many nights, for nearly 4 years. Her cries of anguish and uncontrollable pain even the finest pharmaceuticals couldn't contain. Talk about feeling helpless. I am very grateful to the kind nurses through Hospice. They were on the phone with me quite often in the middle of the night desperately trying to help however they could. It wasn't their first rodeo, that's for sure.

She would be loaded up on enough pharmaceuticals to kill half of a drug rehab clinic with no relief. Finally they started giving us the heavy hitters that pretty much made her semi-comatose. It was better than watching the person you love scramble and squirm on the floor trying to stifle a scream.

Most times I would just sit on the bed next to her and talk. I don't know if she could hear me or not, it didn't matter. Somehow I know she knew I was there. I mostly told her stories about the animals, God knows we had a few. I also would read some of her favorite Bible verses, wet her dry lips with some water or put some chap-stick on them (she hated chapped lips), and I administered the liquid pain medications.

Once she went pretty much comatose, the doctor said I could probably stop giving her the pain medication. I asked, " Probably? Does that mean she can't feel the pain anymore or does it mean that she is just unable to audibly let me know?" He said "it's difficult to know 100%.".

I also asked about withdrawals from the heavy duty pain medications, "do I just stop her cold turkey and she won't feel the withdrawals either?" Again he said "it's hard to be sure 100%." Then I asked "What might she feel or what could happen?" He said "her heart rate might go crazy and she could have a heart attack." I asked him if that was painful and would she feel it? He said "heart attacks can be excruciatingly painful." Whether or not that would happen to her, he said "it was hard to be sure 100%".

Another one of those gut twisting decisions. What is the right choice? Would the heart attack, if it came, take her home early and we could be done with all of this? I figured she had endured enough pain, conscious or unconscious.

I decided to keep giving her the pain medications. I just pulled back her lip a little bit and poured it between the inside of her mouth and teeth then massaged it in until it absorbed. I wanted her to at least be comfortable when she took her last breath. I'll never know if I made the right choice. Just another decision you have to let go of when this is all said and done.

Her last breath was coming any time now. I had asked the hospice nurse what the strange gurgling sound was coming from her throat? She said, "Oh that, that's the death rattle," it usually means that death is knocking at the door and that the person usually signs out within about 48 hours or so.

About a week before she physically left my life forever, even though she was more or less comatose, were these noises she was making that sounded like she was battling demons or some sort of evil entity. It was almost as if Satan was pulling on her soul. The dramatic sounds she was making were beyond your standard nightmare. This went on for 3 or 4 nights and then all of the sudden this tranquil and serene calm came over her. Her breathing mellowed and just a peace about the way she looked, if that makes any sense.

It was almost as if she was being tempted or forced against her will to go somewhere she didn't want to go. I told you before how stubborn she was. She was a strong woman awake, or asleep in a coma, if she didn't want to go somewhere, she wasn't going. Whatever or whoever this strange entity was that she was doing battle with, of course, they or it eventually lost! I wasn't too worried or surprised about "her" losing. I knew who she had backing her up and He doesn't lose the ones that belong to Him, and she definitely belonged to Him. The woman God had so graciously loaned to me for a good percentage of my life was going home.

The last 6 months were probably the most difficult, but I guess that should be expected. She would be up at all hours of the night wanting to do something because she couldn't sleep. The sleeping drugs weren't working anymore.

I don't know how many nights I had to supervise her because she wanted to have a go in the hot tub at 3:30 in the morning or re-arrange the bookshelf in the living room. She also attempted various things in the office and tried to be helpful. She tried to make lists of things she thought we needed but her handwriting at this point was sadly about the level of a 3 year old and totally illegible, the worst part being that on some level, she knew it. She would try with all her might to make those letters legible, but for naught.

That really made her sad, here was this very intelligent, very successful, happy and well organized woman who kept my life and business organized besides her own that couldn't even write the word "apple" legibly.

Her late night, early morning meanderings were like trying to keep an eye on your toddler, doing your best to make sure they didn't hurt themselves. Regardless, it was really hard to get any meaningful sleep.

Of course she didn't want my supervision. I think she wanted to feel like she was still capable of being independent one last time or two. I tried to keep my distance and lurk in the shadows but she was pretty much out of it by then. Such a sweet and innocent demeanor, very childlike. It was really hard to tell her no honey, "I haven't slept in 3 or 4 nights."

I hated myself for having to say no so often. We would be at the grocery store or Costco or something and she would walk by a freshly baked cake or cookies. I'd be over looking at the fruits and vegetables or something related to the cancer diet as usual. She would eagerly glance over at me with her kid in the candy store, beautiful smile and hold up the freshly baked cookies. She had that pleading, childlike, innocent question written all over her face like, daddy, please! It tore out a piece of my heart when I had to say no honey, you can't have sugar, especially refined sugar.

It felt like my heart was bleeding inside my chest. She just wanted to savor the sweet taste of some freshly baked cookies or something, the smell of something in this life that reminded her of better days. Maybe it would be for the last time, I certainly didn't know. Would it really hurt her chance for recovery or were we beyond her chances for recovery? Would it have really have been harmful if I melted from that smile like I wanted to do and said "Okay". Was I being overly strict? That still hurts today, I can still see the look on her face.

I really got sick of having to play the daily role of the strict doctor/professional caregiver. I just wanted to make her happy and make her smile whenever I could. I hated always feeling like her jailer. I hated having to give her the medical reason why I had to say no. I wasn't a doctor, I wasn't some highly trained, nutritional, cancer professional. I was still in school, so to speak. Why is all this being put on me? Why do I have to be the bad guy all the time? I really wanted to be an "anything to make her happy" husband again.

I'm just a woodworker/artist/firefighter/craftsman I guess and now I'm supposed to be this alternative cancer specialist. The pressure was debilitating, too bad for me that I didn't have time for a breakdown. It was a hard rough road that ended up a failure. I just hope she knows how much I loved her and was only being who I was because I so much wanted to save her.

After a long night, I would head out early in the morning to feed the horses, (Rebel, Buddy and Sister), the ducks, the chickens, Little Napoleon, the Banty rooster, Penny the pea hen, Pickles the pig, Jethro the goat, (Dakota-Leone (Dakota), Tuscon the terrible (Tuscon) and Maverick the big brown happy dog, our

Rhodesian Ridgebacks), Ellie and Annabelis Horribilis (Annabelle) the basset hounds, Lacey, Kiko, Pumpkin and Squeaks the cat pack and of course Diego the evil green bird, the doctor of destruction and unbelievable, bone crushing finger pain.

That was the highlight of my day, I got to go clean up horse poop and make sure all the furry kids had feed, clean bedding, and water. In the middle of winter I constructed and stacked up hay bales in the shape of an igloo for the pig. It kept Pickles the pig warm at night with the snow on the ground. We referred to it as the pigloo. The animals were all great therapy for me but best of all they were all good listeners, and I had some good stories I needed to get out of my head. I think they knew something was hurting in my spirit.

I can't tell you how many times I would come back in the house with my heart pounding rapidly, ready to jump out 0f my chest wondering if this was it. Would I look in the bedroom this time and she would be gone?

I cautiously stopped in the hall each time and peered into the bedroom to see if the blankets were moving. Was she breathing? Hard to tell sometimes with 3 Rhodesian Ridgebacks, a Bassett Hound or 2 and 2 or 3 cats all camped out on the bed with her along with a Bible or two opened to her favorite verses.

I don't know if I was being selfish for not wanting her to go. We had been together and in love for like 30 years. Of course we had our moments of confusion and doubt, but in the end the bond we had for so long erased any transgressions in our relationship. I couldn't remember what life was like without her in it, I guess I didn't want to find out.

In the beginning it was really just cruel. Not only were we trying to get past the shock of it all but, the chemo treatments were draining and a downright blockbuster, Hollywood horror film.

We all have our own little slant and idea of what chemo can do to you and your body. It is a world unto its own, its hard to describe from my perspective. All I can say is congratulations to any and all who have endured its application, you are stronger than you know and an inspiration of strength to those on the outside looking in.

I had my own issues I was dealing with. Obviously nothing compared to her but so many alternative treatments she would not agree too. It was a challenge at every turn. If only I knew then what I know now, I know she would still be alive. Anyways that's a brief history of my experience with cancer and all that comes with this nightmare from the depths of hell.

...Why Write This Book?...

I promised Janie that I would spend the rest of my life seeking out ways to defeat this life stealing, life changing monster. Man created it, I strongly and vehemently believe it can be destroyed and eradicated completely by natural means, treating the whole body dynamic.

If I could influence 1 person's life for the better and contribute to their recovery in some way, then all the hours, weeks, days, months and years of endless searching, study and gut wrenching decisions would have some sort of profound meaning.

If I could lessen the agony of the unknown and offer some assurance and hope from total despair to 1 individual, I could smile from the depths of my soul and admit that it was all part of a plan larger than I could conceive.

The idea of being able to share such powerful and life changing, possibly life saving information with another human being gives meaning to my existence, to my suffering as I watched her slowly fade away. I can think of no greater, lasting peace and joy than this type of offering, it's why we're here, it has to be.

Below is a list of some of the alternative treatments that have the highest cure rates. Your cancer can be defeated. You need to believe it! God designed our bodies to be healthy and vibrant and free of disease. Our bodies are smart enough to do just that. We just need to give it the equipment it needs to facilitate a miracle.

I believe in breaking everything down to the basics. How did our Creator design our bodies to function. If we were originally designed for perfection, then what has man altered, taken away or added to our physiology and biology that has changed us.

It's kind of like trying to restore a classic car to its former glory. It isn't worth much with after market parts and modifications. Restore it to all original condition, polish and clean all the original parts to make them like new again and it is nearly priceless. We need to restore our body to its former glory and original design.

As difficult as it may be for many men and women to digest with all the phenomenal technical advances everywhere you turn but, the fact of the matter is, we cannot and should not try and improve on God's ultimate and original design. We just need to find a way to restore our bodies to its original, factory crated, mint condition.

We have somewhere between 50-100 trillion cells in our bodies (the exact number is still up for debate or they lost count or something) all working together with the intent to keep us thriving. When we have disease and or cancer, some component part of the entire system has malfunctioned. Some organ or cell or group of cells is unable to perform its required duty.

That affects everything down the line. Our bodies are like a factory, if one small, simple component of the process is not working properly, chaos is unleashed and optimal, mainline production is halted or interrupted.

...The Mind Game...

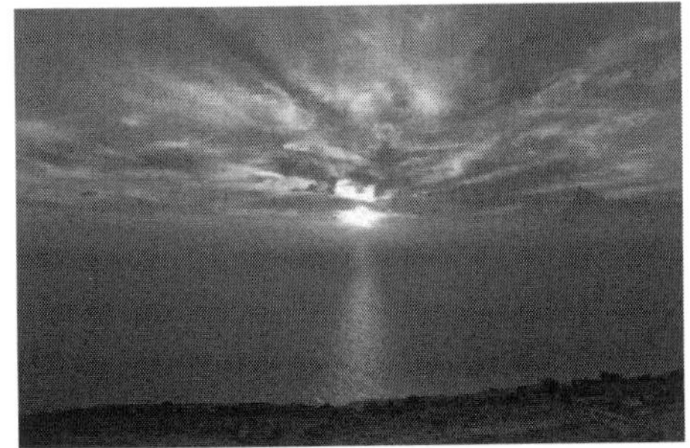

Before you start into any of the modalities or therapies it is vitally important that you put your mind where it needs to be. When you are happy and positive your adrenal glands won't over secrete stress hormones such as cortisol which suppresses your immune system and creates hypertension. It has its place but stress overdoses this hormone.

With a happy, positive outlook your brain secretes neuropeptides, these are the "I'm happy" hormones that communicate directly with the glands of your endocrine system, activating your natural, innate, internal healing response. A 2 thousand year old Chinese medical text, Internal Medicine Classic states, "If one maintains an undisturbed spirit within, no disease will occur."

It works along the same lines as the placebo effect. The subtle hormonal changes that are stimulated by the mind and or the brain are extraordinary. When a patient is given a sugar pill and told that this is an incredible, new, proven miracle pill that will cure their disease, the patient becomes so happy and hopeful that their own innate healing response is activated and they completely recover.

This is not tree-hugger, spiritual delusion or who haw. This is a scientifically proven, indisputable fact. Get your mind where it needs to be! You are a walking miracle, you are incredibly powerful and your body will react to your thought processes. This is just a bump in the road, a lesson along life's indiscriminate encounters.

Of course conventional medicine and the pharmaceutical companies will dismiss this proven fact and categorize it as pure, unadulterated lunacy at best. In their humble opinion their pill or drug is far superior to any perceived sugar pill, placebo or incredibly worthless thought process .

Your mental outlook has a huge impact on the effectiveness of any therapy or treatment. You will severely limit the healing capabilities of your body if you are holding onto grief, anger, fear, loss, low self-esteem, doubt, denial, resentment, paranoia, cynicism or, just an all around pessimistic attitude toward life and your chances for overcoming this diagnosis. It is time to let it go.

The 2 greatest and most important issues you need to absolutely deal with immediately are systemic constipation and your current state of mind. Believe me the game is won or lost in your head. In fact, a doctor in Germany has scientific proof that tragic and immense loss or worry is the precursor to any and all disease.

There is a great deal of scientific evidence confirming the fact that many cancers occur after an exceptionally stressful or tragic life event. The loss of a child, the loss of a spouse, parent, sibling or the loss of a close personal friend are a few events that puncture the lining of our hearts and clearly reveal, through the use of CT scans, abnormal activity in certain areas of the brain.

A Dr. Ryke Geerd Hamer, M.D. investigated the personal histories of his cancer patients and found that they had all suffered from some sort of life altering, tragic event. Dr. Hamer's research illustrated the very close biological relationship between the psyche and the brain and the direct interrelationship with the organs and tissues of the human body.

Dr. Hamer came to name these extraordinary findings "The Five Biological Laws of the New Medicine." These new findings put a completely new spin on the causes, development and healing processes of disease. Dr. Hamer was able to detect and diagram activity in the brain directly relating to certain body parts and organs.

Dr. Hamer concluded that every disease, including cancer, is regulated from its own definitive area in the brain and is tied to a very distinct and identifiable, "conflict shock" in your life.

Unfortunately for Dr. Hamer, these new discoveries conflicted with the status quo of conventional medicine. Dr. Hamer presented these new findings to the proper medical authorities at the university in Germany where he worked. He was then asked to renounce his findings even though there were over 30 scientific studies by independent and other professional associates verifying his hypothesis.

Because he refused to renounce his findings, the renewal of his contract at the university was denied. In 1986 his medical license was revoked for not adhering to the principles and doctrines of standard medicine.

Because of his revolutionary studies and his refusal to comply with the medical establishment, Dr. Hamer is currently living in exile in Spain where he continues his research. He has been harassed and persecuted by the German and French authorities for over 25 years.

Dr. Hamer named this stressful event in someone's life DHS (Dirk Hamer Syndrome) in honor of the son he lost in 1978. DHS is characterized by an unanticipated, stressful and tragic, life event. He concluded that this event not only takes it's toll on us psychologically but biologically too.

After analyzing thousands of CT scans and comparing them to a patients past histories, he discovered that the moment this DHS event occurs, it impacts a specific area in the brain causing a lesion that is visible on the scan. The affected brain cells then communicate this shock to a corresponding organ. This in turn responds with a particular and predictable alteration.

This ties into the research showing how certain areas of the brain are preprogramed to respond to conflicts or threats to our survival. Other areas of the brain are programmed to other survival basics like breathing, eating and reproduction.

Without getting too far into the science behind his discoveries, this all tracks back to the ultimate power of our minds and our thoughts. Tumors can develop from these stress induced, every-day, "conflict shocks."

An example would be lung cancer from the "death-fright conflict" of not being able to breathe. The lung alveoli, which regulate our breathing, start to multiply in order to survive the death panic you created in your mind of not being able to breathe. This in turn can initiate the growth of a tumor.

Breast cancer can be tied to a mother-child worry conflict. If a child is seriously injured or ill the breast gland cells begin to multiply from a preprogrammed signal in the brain to produce more milk for the suffering offspring. This "conflict shock" stress phase initiates an age old biological function in it's attempt to speed up potential healing. This preprogrammed biological response of proliferating cells, forms a tumor.

Dr Hamer differentiates between the actions of the "Old brain" controlled areas and organs and the "New brain" controlled areas. "Old brain" controlled areas seem to generate tumor growth during the active phase of the conflict whereas the "New brain," in the active phase of the conflict responds with cell degeneration and necrosis of the biologically corresponding organ tissues.

I just wanted to give you some concrete scientific research to back up what I am trying to get across. How you deal with conflict directly affects all aspects of your life. It can and will determine whether or not you succumb to disease, and it will affect your ability to heal and restore yourself through your immune system. You can't overlook this huge component, you can't rely solely on the treatment, you have to be in the game and you have to be in it to win. It's called "The brain game".

Write down daily affirmations of healing and of hope and of miracles. When you program your mind with positive affirmations on a consistent basis your subconscious mind will go to work on bringing that thought process to fruition and to your reality.

This is the single most important thing you need to do before you start any treatment. I know it is an immense mind game especially with what you are facing, but it is beyond crucial for your recovery.

The power of written words are astonishing. Be sure and write down some very powerful affirmations. Make copies and keep them in your car, in your house, in your purse, next to the toilet. Meditate on them. Recite them diligently, daily, multiple times. Make it a habit.

In fact, if you want to see first hand the power of the written word and your thoughts, try this experiment. Cook up a standard serving of rice, I know, this is getting weird, stay with me. After you are finished cooking the rice, take 2 different containers, the closer each portion of the experiment is identical the better, place ½ of your cooked rice in 1 container and the other ½ in the other container.

Now write some happy, grateful words on 1 container and write some hateful, angry words on the other container. Something like; I love you, your beautiful, I'm so grateful on one container, and I hate you, your despicable and your ugly or something on the other container. I'm sure you can think of some good words.

Place the containers somewhere where they will be subjected to the same environment. Maybe on a dresser or something. Each day or a couple of times a day, pick up the container and speak the words and mean it, be grateful for what this food does for your body. Watch what happens in a week or two. And no I'm not insane, just a test please. You can even do this experiment without speaking the words, just let the words do their thing.

...Clearing the Debris...

Once you get your mindset where it needs to be and you have written out your daily affirmations, its time to work on the blood and your organs of elimination. Your blood is the central character in all processes in the body. It delivers nutrients to our cells including oxygen, helps build and replace worn out parts and carries away our cellular waste.

Your lymphatic system performs a job similar to your blood. You have approximately 3 times more lymphatic fluid in your body than blood and around 6-700 lymph glands. The lymphatic system also clears toxins and acid wastes from the blood and your tissues.

Your heart is the pump that moves your blood throughout your body, your lymphatic system relies on movement. It has no pump, although it is just as crucial as your blood in delivery and removal of nutrients and toxic debris.

This is one of the reasons why exercise of some sort is so healthful and so extremely important for body functioning. Most do not address this critical component. Exercise or body movement facilitates movement of lymphatic fluid, otherwise, it can become stagnant and quite literally, constipated. It can't move unless you move, get up, do something, turn the T.V. off. And no, don't use the remote, get up and turn it off.

One of the best exercises to accomplish this movement is rebounding. That is the small round trampoline (around 3 feet diameter) you set up and use at home. This simple exercise of gently jumping up and down accelerates the movement of lymphatic fluid and greatly enhances the efficiency in clearing out congested areas.

Any type of exercise will influence this movement but rebounding is very beneficial especially when facing a life threatening illness. It is crucial that this delivery and removal system be functioning at peak proficiency. Depending on the severity of your condition, even mild exercise like walking or any other consistent movement will help to open up and distribute the flow of lymphatic fluid.

...What To Start Thinking About...

Wow, what a ride! Now that I have been studying this affliction for well over 10 years, night and day, where in the world do you start if you have just been diagnosed with some form of cancer?

Before you jump into any type of natural or alternative treatment you need to make sure your organs of elimination are operating at peak efficiency. You need to give this some serious, primary consideration.

I was so scrambled with panic at first that I was all over the place. I may have touched on some of the best modalities out there but, I didn't understand the importance of eliminating the toxic debris once one of these protocols was implemented and started to work.

In my opinion, and it's only my opinion. Number 1: make sure you talk to your physician. Number 2: I believe you need to examine your life and your diet. What have you been eating? Make a list of your average daily food consumption and variety of foods, your average week too.

How much is processed? How much is cooked in a microwave, fried in oil? How else are you cooking your food? How much is raw, organic etc.? What has been your average ratio of cooked to raw foods for the last 5 years? You really need to switch to the 80% raw, 20% lightly cooked ratio. I know you have been eating the other way around, haven't you?

What prescription medications are you taking? For how long? What over the counter medications? How much? How many? How long have you been taking them and what's in them that might be harmful? What supplements or vitamins do you take? Same thing, how much? How many? How long? Are they whole, unadulterated, natural vitamins or are they man-made, isolated, stand alone, synthetic supplements?

What are or have you been exposed to, growing up, at work, at home? Was or is any of it potentially toxic? Do you take any kind of laxative to go to the bathroom or are you really regular? Is your poop a good consistency and amount? Sorry, just keeping it real.

I know, maybe a little to personal but, How is your marriage? Are you happy? Are you generally a happy person? Any major problems with your children? Any enduring grief you are holding onto? What other emotional issues are you dealing with? Are you overly stressed? Do you have any hobbies or any other things that you enjoy, activities that make you smile and laugh and do you take part in them regularly? Are you an excessive worrier? Are your finances making you crazy? When was your last vacation?

Try and figure out what may have contributed or is contributing to your current situation and deal with it however that has to happen. You are looking for a long term recovery. It's time to remove as many negatives and unresolved issues as you can. You have to get your head screwed on straight.

I really can't say all these things too many times. To help get your mind straight you might want to try to just keep dwelling on the placebo effect. That's at least well documented. Most people have themselves or have someone close to them that's been fooled by some sort of placebo.

It doesn't have to involve a sugar pill. It just has to be something we thought was real or true that made a change occur, whether it was real or not. Just thinking that it was, is usually enough. It's real and it's magical. Believe it or not your mind alone could cure your affliction if it was conditioned and experienced enough. It all comes back to your Faith. Find it! Maybe its time to finally start that meditation or yoga or Qigong class you've been talking about, you know, the one you keep putting off. Don't give me that look, you know who you are!

...Constipation and Cancer...

They say that constipation along with malnutrition kills more people every year than any form of disease or accidental death. More than any other affliction combined, worldwide.

Consuming a diet that has nowhere near the nutrition needed to sustain a healthy body eventually gets your attention. We then compound that problem with our inability to move what we did consume out through our large intestine. The result is constipation and the initiation of cancer and disease.

Our bodies were designed to breakdown our meals, absorb whatever nutrition was in that meal and discard the leftovers. In other words, take what we need and let our bowels and other organs of elimination do what they were designed to do, get rid of the trash.

That is the basic premise of our design and our bowels are the largest organ of elimination besides the skin. We do have many other components that contribute to the removal of leftover metabolic debris.

Some of the other components would be our arteries, veins, capillaries and lymphatic system. The quality and efficiency of these systems also rely on the quality and availability of nutrients in what we eat. What we eat determines how effectively and efficiently these systems perform.

We typically associate constipation with our lower bowels. Whether you understand it or not, your arteries, veins, capillaries and lymphatic system can also become constipated. After all, what we eat either feeds the system or gets left behind in the form of deposits and plaques. So, putting it into perspective, what we really have is systemic constipation, whole body constipation. Nothing is moving out and clearing the system as well as it could and should be.

We all know that once disease is diagnosed, a particular organ is usually isolated and labeled as the culprit and blamed for the breakdown. The truth is that there is usually a reason why this organ malfunctioned or broke down in the first place. It was not given what it needed to survive and thrive either from a restricted or an obstructed delivery system.

So in essence, it wasn't per say a weak liver or heart or whatever, although, some specific organ or part will get the blame in all this. Liver disease, heart disease, renal failure, bladder irregularities, incontinence etc., you know the list. Your probably taking some form of medication for one of these right now. I know my mother has a plethora of daily prescriptions she takes, 1 for her kidneys, 1 for high blood pressure, 1 for water retention, 1 for hypothyroidism, 1 for indigestion 1 for etc. etc..

I guess isolated organ damage and or failures are a good thing for the economy. That way we create specialists for every single part of the body. It keeps the medical schools busy brimming with post graduate, extended layover, specialist training classes.

Wow, what a concept. What if instead of specialist training for a particular organ or body part class, they taught how to improve the overall condition of the whole body through diet and the elimination of leftover metabolic waste? What if they taught how to super charge the immune system through the fuel we feed it (diet) so disease didn't have a chance to damage an organ or body function in the first place. Why? Where's the profits in that? Where's the profit in telling your patients to make sure they eat their broccoli and brussel sprouts?.

The simple fact is that most of the time it is a malfunctioning delivery system that created the bad organ. A constipated, systemic delivery system is many times the culprit. Find the damaged delivery system, fix it, repair it and a good majority of the time the malfunctioning organ will revive and restore itself. No preservatives or added food colorings, all natural restoration. The best part being it will do it without drugs or surgery. Good for you, bad for the doctors.

What I'm trying to say is that sometimes it is not necessarily the isolated organ that failed. The delivery system that you fed with an improper diet failed, and that delivery system failed to feed the organ what it required. Get it. It's really common sense 101. It just seems so logical, why does it turn into something so complicated?.

If you own a gas station and the gas isn't coming out of the pump when you pull the handle, do you work on the pump or do you look for another reason why the gas isn't coming out? Conventional medicine will typically send you to a pump specialist.

You have to figure out why the fuel isn't coming out of the pump, maybe it is getting to the pump it's just not coming out, why is the pump failing? Maybe the pump isn't the problem. The pump is fine or will be fine. It would appear on the surface to be the problem, after all, it's not pumping gas but, the gas has to get to the pump for it to work, right? Sadly, the pump gets the blame for being broken, so now we need that pump specialist.

Conventional medicine will typically just give you buckets full of gas (drugs) to manually fill the pump. Too many times they will not investigate and diagnose the kink in the hose that feeds the pump. The kink in the hose is the problem, fix the kink and the pump will magically repair itself and start working again. In the meantime, the pump appears to be in need of repair. You will just be wasting your money. Until you fix the kink, the pump will continue to give you that illusion.

Okay back to the issues I needed to give more attention too. Here I go again and I know I say "I can't say it too many times" too many times but, the toxic sludge and acidic wastes need to find their way out of the body. You can't just keep on piling up trash in the corner somewhere, I don't need to explain what will happen if you do. Okay, just 1. Besides the smell, it becomes the perfect breeding ground for pests, flies, maggots and other parasitic bacteria. I know, that was 2 things. Now at least you have a visual.

Of course Janie was on heavy duty pain medication and we all pretty much know what they do to your morning eliminations, if you are able to eliminate at all. I remember trying all sorts of over the counter and natural, herbal supplements. I wasn't really overly focused on the issue, more of a uh oh, you have to go to the bathroom, try this.

Surely this well educated, Holistic/Homeopathic doctor in Reno we went to would have said something to me if it was that critical, right? Believe me, regardless of who is treating you, you need to keep up with any and all aspects of the journey into recovery. No one has all the answers and no one remembers all the details so you have to do your homework. By the way, I'm hoping this book will be a part of your homework.

I didn't realize that moving your bowels consistently with the proper shape, form, color, amount, and that the contents of the movement were so critical. I was too focused on the cures and what to try next. Need to hurry right? This is stage IV, no time for technicalities and the basic bodily functions.

Yes, going to the bathroom was important but I didn't understand or grasp the massively important enormity of being able to consistently go. How else was the many years of chemical sludge going to leave her body. Your bowel movements and systemic constipation are in my opinion the number 1 cause for immediate concern and primary, mandatory action.

If and when one of these natural, alternative treatments started working I guess I just assumed that that was the highlight and I didn't give it much more thought about how this dying or dead cancer debris would get out of the body.

What a huge mistake! I needed to connect all the dots on how the body functioned. The stupid simple basics. We eat, we absorb whatever nutrients were in that food and then we poop out what we didn't need. I needed to take my eyes off of the cure and the joy of remission and or healing and see the overall, big picture or little picture, it seems so simple now. Pretty much those 3 simple steps. Eat, absorb and poop. Give those 3 things the attention they deserve and you won't need to read this book.

I'm writing this E-book so you will not overlook what I did. So you will not get ahead of yourself in panic and the need for a quick result. The body is amazing. Help it according to the way it was designed to function. Don't put your own spin on it, start with the simple basics.

...What Foods To Avoid...

You can start by eliminating all meat and dairy from your diet. All animal based protein sources. Laboratory experiments have confirmed that animal based proteins feed cancer. Also, these foods are the most troublesome and labor intensive for the body to digest and we need the body's energy to focus elsewhere.

Did you know that the pancreas plays a huge role in destroying cancer cells? When the pancreas is too busy breaking down labor intensive foodstuffs it can get overwhelmed. Part of the reason type II diabetes is on the rise. It gets overwhelmed by the artificial, synthetic and animal based foods we devour. We cook almost all of our foods and have destroyed many if not all of our necessary enzymes.

Eating without enzymes is like going to war and sending in an army of tanks, Humvees and a massive platoon of soldiers. Only 1 significant problem, there's no ammunition. They do their best searching around on the ground for any extra rounds and manage to acquire some scraps here and there. They even manage to steal some from the enemy but eventually, they're completely disabled and unable to perform.

Anyway, maybe not the best comparison but, when we eat, the enzymes are the ammunition necessary to complete the mission successfully. Okay, back to the elimination thing. The morning ritual for most. For those of you who are blessed, more than once a day is great as long as your movements are well formed and complete. I know it sounds disgusting but your poop can tell you a lot about what is happening inside of your body. Take a look next time, you know you look. Any worms or other creepy crawlers? Is it black, is it well formed? In other words is it what you would call a quality elimination? That really is another book.

There is a vast network of knowledgeable, natural health related experts that believe and agree that all disease starts in the colon. The efficiency and performance of our intestinal tract is the star of the show and rules what happens in the rest of our body. Because of all the worthless junk food we consume, our intestinal tract and our digestive system is highly overworked and abused on a regular, consistent, and ongoing basis.

You can't dismiss or skim over the clogged up colon issue. Not only do natural health practitioners believe that all disease begins in the gut and colon but many modern day conventional medical practitioners are beginning to support this belief. The list of afflictions directly related to an inefficient digestive system and colon is staggering. Some of the founders of our modern day medical system believe that neurological disorders and even insanity is initiated and caused by digestive system disturbances.

You know that the body can only survive for so long without food. It's the fuel that keeps us running. It's like gas in your car, when you run out of fuel in your car, the car is dead. Same with you, when you run out of fuel, you're more or less dead. You may still be breathing but death is close by.

Every cell, organ, muscle, bone, ligament and tissue relies on fuel to function, period. Simple, basic, life sustaining fuel (food). Then there's the quality of the food. What happens to your car when you put 80 octane fuel in it when it has to have at least 87 octane for everything to perform ? Yes it will chug along on 80 octane but for how long? How long have you been chugging along? How long have you been putting cheap, inadequate, low octane food in your digestive tank? When's the last time you felt amazing, high octane amazing?

There are many different colon cleansing products on the market. Of course they all claim to be the best, all natural, organic formula's available. I'm not going to analyze or bash any of them.

Many are very effective and do help clean out the system. But how thoroughly?

Okay, I won't do another one of my comparisons, but, over the counter laxatives and even powerful herbal colon cleanses typically will not pick up a lifetime of caked on sludge. Some do extremely well but can take to much time time. You may not have that time.

It is an amazing and magical experience, almost nirvana, when you are able to remove and pass that filthy layer of toxic, mucous infested, caked on sludge. The boost to the immune system from the increased bio-availability and absorption of nutrients is phenomenal and beyond belief. Your whole world changes.

You have to submit to the coffee enemas, they are of primary and mandatory importance, especially for a cancer diagnosis. Do not be afraid, just be sure and let your doctor know what you will be doing.

...Who Do You Trust?...

Another point of interest and curiosity is not to believe all the nutritional advice being handed down from your conventional healthcare professional. If by a very narrow chance they actually mention anything about nutrition and diet. The majority will not.

Many times the information they give you is just not as accurate as you would think. I know you are thinking these people went to school and or college and have a piece of paper that says they have all the right answers. If it's taught in school then it must be true, right? If it's in a textbook it's supposed to be a fact. Right? Sad to say that things are not always what they seem. Just think about all the history that has been re-written as more facts become uncovered. The information in textbooks is not infallible and set in stone, nothing is.

In our conventional medical schools, nutrition and diet are barely touched upon, and when it is the people that put together the nutritional and standard diet information have certain special interest groups that influence the facts or what would appear to be the facts.

I'm not saying that these nutritional experts are outright lying to you, I would say they definitely are not. They most assuredly want to help. They are only telling you what they know from what they have been taught in school. That's part of the reason why it takes so long to sort through all the research and documentation. Then you have to decide what relevant research was truly without bias. So much of it is slanted to scratch the backs of some special interest group. It's the same with everything, he who has the gold.

Think of all the new and improved medicines, pharmaceuticals and let's not forget the massively growing vitamin industry. With more and more people taking the latest, greatest, laboratory approved pharmaceutical grade vitamins, you would think that cancer would be getting its butt kicked. Yet, cancer continues to skyrocket out of control!

Thing is, our bodies haven't changed. Our environment and our food has. Our bodies still need the basics. The basics found in nature the way God packaged them. Our bodies don't need some newly discovered, Earth shattering, laboratory created super-charged vitamin. We just need our basic fruits, vegetables and oils grown in and from the Earth. Hopefully grown with naturally decomposed, mineral rich, organic soils, clean water, fresh air and a respectable amount of sunshine.

I know, so much of this stuff was new to me too. Some of it I only just learned as I continue to study. Back in the beginning I didn't have a lot of time to ponder and reflect. Nobody recommended anything, nobody really knew of any alternatives. It was a treat as you go protocol, and we had to start right away. There was no one to talk too. No one to lead us in the right direction. Want to talk about anxious? That was me.

Like I said, I was all over the place. Of course I grew up with the reliance and faith most of us have in our conventional way of medicine. The Holistic/Organic approach didn't hold much promise initially since it was so far out of my comfort zone.

I didn't really have a lot of faith in the possibility that these treatments really worked.

I was old school, die hard, stubborn, and stupid too. Some of them just seemed too simple. There's no way in God's green Earth these could possibly work, could they? If they really worked surely the news would be out. It was out alright, it had just morphed into something obscure. The information that was out there was immediately and covertly controlled by the billionaire elite.

Thank God I always had an open mind, I always wanted to hear the other side of whatever. I liked making my own deductions and decisions armed with the ammunition of truth.

The biggest hurdle for me was believing the conspiracy of the pharmaceutical companies and the medical establishments monopoly over the treatment of cancer. I couldn't grasp the idea of a cover up. Too many people were dying and suffering horrendously. I should know, I had a front row seat.

I guess I was sort of in the crowd that scoffed and joked behind the backs of the so called Herbal/Earthy healers and such. Of course, I also grew up with that re-enforcement from my circle of family and friends that would openly criticize and castigate those damned environmentalist wacko's stirring up trouble again for the more than prestigious conventional establishment.

I think the conventional establishment made up the word conspiracy so that they would have a word they could use to make people feel stupid for believing anything other than mainline politics. You know who I'm talking about, don't you?

Those folks that immediately judge you and label you a conspiracy theorist and then chuckle thinking you're an idiot because you have a differing slant on things. They are the ones that are hopelessly lost and blinded. After you actually start uncovering the reality, you realize that our institutions of good faith and public trust, initially sworn to serve under the motto of "One Nation Under God" have replaced "God" with "Power."

Back when I was growing up, anyone who supported or agreed with the animal rights people, the environmentalists, the save the planet folks and let's not forget those wacky vegetarians, was a numbskull, a halfwit, and a left-wing liberal treehugger. Boy, have I come a long way, I think I'm all of those now, except the numbskull, halfwit and left-wing liberal.

Now I'm proud to say I'm a vegetarian, animal rights supporter, save the planet promoter, environmentalist and a treehugger. I'm not an extremist but I do have a great amount of love and respect for anything connected to the environment, the Earth and our survival.

It's amazing how incredibly intelligent and committed these environmental soldiers of the Earth really are. I'm talking about the people that have uncovered and solved the conspiracies, know the truth and truly care about changing what corporate America is doing to our future and our childrens future environment. This is really all about slick cars, massive yachts, multiple homes and all the other exorbitant luxuries money can buy. Seems that everyone has their price.

As for me, I had always been a major animal lover so making that part of the change was easy, and I always had respect for people and the environment, it's either a part of who you are or it's not. The environment thing changed for me drastically when I made the move to Wyoming and experienced what a real ecosystem and a pristine forest was really all about.

It is equally amazing through education, research and logic how so many truths have inherited the title of conspiracy. It's just a word used to blanket the truth. So many far reaching and at one time, completely ridiculous conspiracies have proven to be undeniably true.

My earlier growing pains with eyes wide shut have now been opened to the endless possibilities and magic of Nature. How to enjoy it and utilize it's infinite healing applications and weapons of mass disease destruction.

Recently, I heard from an acquaintance who has a friend dying of cancer. They both, through their own speculative reasoning, believe that alternative cancer therapies and herbal medicine are conspiracies against conventional medicine. He has been given up by conventional means and won't even consider alternatives. Hmmmmm.

It would seem the conventional medical establishment has done an exemplary job of blinding the people. Their marketing of the dangers and absolute stupidity of even considering alternative therapies as a viable option in the treatment of cancer has made it's mark. Unfortunately, it's applications will remain an absurdity in the minds of many.

By the way, what does alternative medicine have to gain in a conspiracy against conventional medicine? I'm not sure, seems there would be much more money and incentive the other way around. Some will never believe, and sadly they will die supporting their allegiance to orthodox medicine. It all comes down to your education and what you know.

I spent 16, 17, 18, sometimes 19 hours a day reading or researching online, offline and by my own personal experiences. Sorting through the clutter, searching for the answers, that was my life.

I'm so grateful I had alternatives to turn to when the conventional monarchy had nothing left to offer us. Even being completely ignorant, I at least had to try and, bless her heart, she gave it all she had, too. We thought we made it. We thought we had defeated this monster. I didn't know what I was going to do if she went away.

Surely someone would help me gather all the pieces of my life back together, financially, mentally and physically if she happened to lose her battle. If only I had the friends she had. I lost it all, everything. I'm not saying I didn't have amazing friends, I absolutely did. But nobody can even fathom the anguish and pain that was to follow.

It really is hard enough to watch your spouse suffer for nearly 4 years and then lose the battle. I lost my wife, and by my own stupidity thinking I could save her, lost the house and my business. The Trifecta of life. What a slam. Talk about getting hit up side the head. Oh well, we all have our defeats.

I figure there must be something positive coming from all this. I hope that what you are reading is a part of that positive, I hope this book breaks through the deeply ingrained, deeply conditioned conspiracy barrier. I pray that you can open your mind far enough to see the trees. They are real and they are beautiful. I hope and pray everyday that this information blesses someone.

I did have full time company during and after the drama was over, and I thank God everyday for my always present, always loyal, companion and dog, Mr. Maverick. Janie knew she might not survive this ordeal and she wanted to make sure I had a loyal friend, a nonjudgmental, constant companion to help me through the shock of being alone for the first time in 30 years. So she picked out the most amazing, full time, around the clock company anyone could ever ask for, a Rhodesian Ridgeback named Maverick.

After taking care of a loved one for nearly 4 years, non-stop, I needed a living, breathing, constant companion that needed to be taken care of. It was the only thing I was accustomed to doing for the last 4 years, care giving. I needed something or someone that relied on me for life.

We didn't have any children, although we had tried. Somebodies wiring wasn't firing on all cylinders. We were looking into adoption, sadly, just before her diagnosis. Mainly because of the amazing array of animals we had on the ranch. We figured we needed a child or two to enjoy all this love that emanated from every part of the property.

So, with no kids, I'd be lost without someone or something to take care of at this point. I had my routine, and you know how hard routines are to break. My amazing Rhodesian Ridgeback, Maverick, was a consistent and constant part of my recovery.

I had someone that would listen when I needed to talk or just hang out with me and watch a movie when I felt like staring at a box, no strings attached. Maybe a little strange for you folks that are non dog connoisseurs but it worked for me.

There were some emotional issues to overcome being the amount of time the dogs spent hanging out with Janie while she was sick. It was gut wrenching when Maverick and Ellie, (the basset hound), would hear a car pulling up the drive and get excited thinking their Mommy was finally coming back home. I think Maverick still wonders why she left and never came back. I don't know how I would have fared without him.

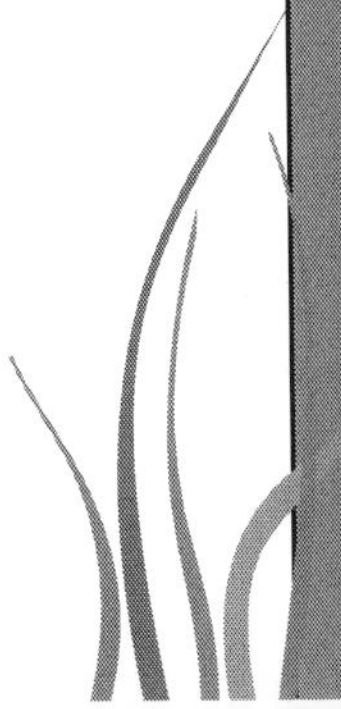

Chapter 2

Fasting

> "Everyone has a doctor in him or her; we just have to help it in its work. The natural healing force within each one of us is the greatest force in getting well. Our food should be our medicine. Our medicine should be our food. But to eat when you are sick, is to feed your sickness."
>
> —Hippocrates

The Bible quotes these words from Jesus; "Renew yourselves and fast, for I tell you truly, except you fast, you shall never be freed from the power of Satan and all diseases that come from Satan."

One of the best ways to clear out your colon is with juice fasting. Consuming nothing but liquid, cleansing, fruit and vegetable juices frees up the digestive system to do its job. It's like giving your digestive system a vacation.

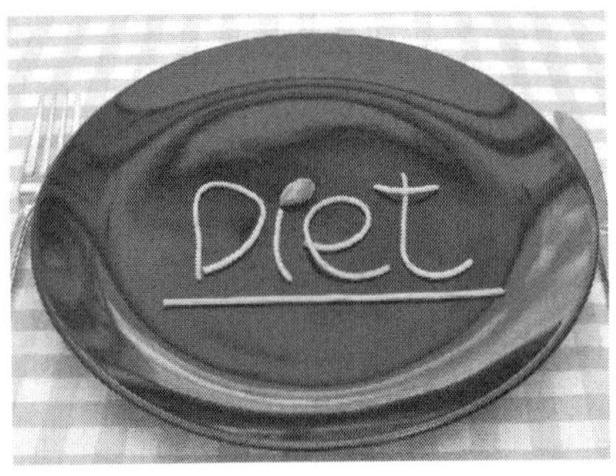

Your body knows what to do, believe me. Your body knows it is sick. Your body knows there is a breakdown somewhere. Give it a chance to do just that, repair the breakdown. Our bodies have a built in, innate program that initiates an internal cleansing.

Our bodies are constantly at work distributing oxygen and nutrients to our cells, feeding our cells. They are also constantly removing spent fuel from our metabolic processes and taking out the trash or removing foreign, toxic, leftover debris from that process.

With juice fasting you more or less bypass the digestive process. It passes straight through. The nutrients will be absorbed into the blood from your intestinal tract and the rest will be sent where it needs to go to be eliminated.

Juice fasting is becoming more and more popular. More people, especially those on the SAD (Standard American Diet) diet, need to be more aware of the condition of their intestines. At least they should be. Every other person, actually, just about everyone you talk to has a problem with constipation.

It is so incredibly crucial to our health being that we are bombarded daily with way too many additives, chemicals, foods grown in man-made, inorganic soils, preservatives, artificial colorings, nitrites, nitrates and foods that have been genetically altered and or irradiated. Of course this is all done for our "safety".

It could even be considered a conspiracy. If you think about the damage done to our bodies with all these foreign substances, a grass roots, massively, busting at the seams business was formed. The sick industry, it grows bigger and bigger every year and business is booming. Our economy would fall on its face if people were healthy, sad, but that's the reality.

Any ideas why we are so sick? Are you constipated? The majority of Americans are severely constipated. I have a friend that poops pellets or rocks every other day yet continues to eat lifeless, dead, de-vitalized fast food. He has hemorrhoids from constantly straining to get anything out and a massively distended abdomen. I have a good guess as to what the distention is from. Incomplete evacuations and impacted fecal matter.

What I don't understand is why do we wait till a major life threatening illness strikes before we wake up? When it's that obvious it boggles the mind. Some people are just plain overweight, everywhere. Some people have a huge accumulation of isolated fat in their abdomen.

It is almost always a constipation problem that needs to be immediately addressed. Please do not wait. It's like driving around on a bald tire, sure it's holding air for right now but eventually it's going to blow. What if your going 70 miles an hour when it blows???

When toxic matter becomes trapped in our large intestine the normal peristaltic action, the movement of the muscle that pushes whatever waste towards its exit point, shuts down or becomes severely impaired. It will, sooner, rather than later, shut down completely if you are relying on OTC laxatives. This particular way of dealing with it will initiate an early demise.

Many have seen pictures of what results from this peristaltic shutdown. More and more undigested matter begins accumulating and becomes impacted. Patients on a thorough colon cleanse or enema regimen have reported passing a black, plastic like mucus lining that has taken on the shape of their interior, intestinal wall.

Most people address constipation with an over the counter laxative to create a breakthrough where at least something is able to pass. This does nothing to remedy this trapped black mucus or to revive peristaltic movement or muscle action. Over the counter laxatives actually kill this vital muscle and the body will become dependent on this form of laxative. It's good for the economy though. You become a customer for life.

The main purpose of fasting is to remove this mucus and systemic constipation from the body and its tissues. Some people describe it as being reborn when this black impacted mass finds its way out.

The longer you commit to a fasting program and diet, the more healing and the more cleansing you will experience. It is said that there are no incurable diseases only people who believe they cannot be cured.

Fasting is critical to our overall health and longevity. The Taoist principle of 'wu-wei' means noninterference or not doing. This not doing, meaning no solid food or abstinence from food, initiates and awakens the body's most powerful healing and cleansing responses.

We are supposed to learn from our surroundings, from nature and from the animals who have a remarkable innate sense. A sense many times greater than our own. Nearly, if not all animals refuse to eat when they are ill.

I'm sure many of you have experienced your dog or cat not eating. You get worried and go out and buy a steak or some hamburger to cook. A nice home cooked meal for them in an attempt to get them to eat, right?

Wrong, don't do that! They are not eating for a reason. They are fasting. They have an innate sense of what needs to happen to bring about recovery. We need to learn something from that.

Many ancient tribes from around the world still practice fasting. They have sick houses where those that are ill go to recover. Here they rest comfortably and abstain from all solid food until they recover their health.

Modern day medical practitioners dismiss fasting as an old and outdated resource primitive cultures used that didn't have access to the pharmaceutical drugs commonly prescribed for each and every ill known to man. How lucky were they?

Modern day alternative medical practitioners are producing great success stories using fasting when all other conventional attempts have failed. Recent scientific research and clinical studies have proven conclusively that fasting and caloric restriction are the keys to enhanced health and a longer, more vibrant life.

A scientific report was released in 1986 where laboratory mice were severely restricted on their dietary intake. Those that were restricted lived far longer than did the mice that were allowed to eat as much and as often as they wished.

Some of the pioneers of fasting like Dr. Norman Walker, Paul Bragg and V.E. Irons lived to nearly 100 years plus and remained active and vibrant until the day they died.

What if at 50-60 years of life you were only halfway there? Some say V.E. Irons would have lived to 120+ if fate had not intervened with a tragic car accident.

V.E. Irons was a huge advocate in the use of enemas. He practiced it religiously and nearly completely cured a severe, irreversible degenerative condition in his spine. Doctors gave him little hope for a normal life without major medical intervention, and also very limited mobility. He chose nature and the infamous "Colema Board," the home convenience enema board people can easily use to administer enemas at home. Fun for the whole family!

Your body is fully aware of what it needs to do. When your digestive enzymes are free of the labor of digestion, they go to work digesting toxic buildup and acidic debris. Since no new wastes are being ingested, the body initiates its own life force of restoration.

This is where your colon and other organs of elimination need to be functioning at their peak efficiency. If the body is naturally initiating this cleansing process, this dead, dying matter needs to find its way out.

The fasting also triggers the release and production of human growth hormones which, start the work of rejuvenating tissue and vital functions in the body.

Our normal reduction of this hormone as we age is one of the main causes of age related degenerative conditions, including how long we live and how much life force and energy we are able to create and sustain.

Fasting has been around for thousands of years. It only makes sense don't you think? Our bodies are so intricately designed where trillions of cells are communicating non stop, without any outside help from the medical establishment.

It only stands to reason that a machine as miraculous as the human body would have a built in garbage in garbage out system of repair.

The problem is we are addicted to fast and easy and with a fast food joint on every corner of the universe, it's really hard to avoid, right? We can't even buy gas anymore without a plethora of snacks and chemical laced chips and jerky's to tempt our weakened resolve.

They put such well thought out, laboratory tested, addictive chemicals in our food, we are continually and habitually lusting for more. They really work hard to target the kids with all the child directed marketing gimmicks. It certainly seems to be working, to hell with our health and the health of our children, pass me the chips and the chemical dip.

I recently purchased a real, 100%, grass fed and organically grown, Angus beef hamburger for one of my stepdaughters. She couldn't eat it, she thought it tasted horrible. She was too accustomed to the chemical, sugar laced, processed fast food, are you sure this is really beef, burger.

If you think about it, targeting the kids and hooking them early on bad for you food secures a lifelong customer. Everybody wins except the kids down the road. The medical establishment keeps busy and will continue to keep busy as these children age and start manifesting the diseases that come with eating an anti-nutritious diet. What happened to "you eat what's on your plate and you eat whatever everyone else is eating or go hungry"? That worked for me growing up. It would seem to me there are far too many modern day kids that have never learned the meaning of grateful, of having a plate full of food period.

One more thing while I'm on the subject. Why is it that so many children dictate to their parents what they will eat. They wine and they cry because they want to go to their favorite fast food joint.

Many parents I know even cook different meals for different children. Johnny won't eat that and Julie only likes this and Jackie doesn't like that. OMG. Since when are children smart enough to make such enormous decisions about what their body needs to survive? Isn't that why we are the parents? To protect them from harmful foodstuffs. I know, we're tired and it's just easier to give in and give them what they want.

Sad part being that we are conditioning them for their future habits. Yes we're tired but it comes back to bite us in the butt. They become so addicted to worthless food and candy, they carry that addiction into their adult life, besides creating a living hell at home for the parents deciding how and what to cook for each child. Ok sorry, a little off track but these children are our next generation of infirmities.

It's sad that so many simple, basic, no-brainer traditions like fasting have been laid aside to make room for the supreme authority and decisiveness of the food corporations and the medical establishment. But then again, promoting something like fasting isn't profitable. It is not patentable. It's a worthless myth sold by the purveyors and instigators of quackery that has been passed down through antiquity, yes?

That last line, passed down through antiquity, doesn't that have a message in it. If it was a worthless, silly, meaningless part of medicine way back then wouldn't it have died and burnt itself out a long time ago? I mean, how long can something totally without merit hold up?

Does it matter that, Aristotle, Plato, Socrates and other historically respected Greek philosophers did their best to try and set the standard for our Western culture and style by fasting regularly.

Many of these philosophers even required their students to fast before offering their highest and most honorable insights and enlightenment's. They were convinced that it improved and elevated their overall physical health and mental capacity.

The ancient sages were quite aware of the connection between the body and the mind. They knew way back then that whatever pollutes the body, pollutes and manifests in the mind.

They knew that toxic blood and other toxic bodily fluids not only invited microbes, viruses and disease, but that this poisoning of the body degraded and destroyed the human spirit.

The Bible actually mentions fasting 74 times. Early in the twentieth century, the Dead Sea Scrolls were discovered and a most remarkable document was found, written in Aramaic. It was later, in 1937, translated into English under the title "The Essene Gospel of Peace." It details some of the most well known and important healings that Jesus performed.

The teachings in this Gospel are vitally important to the health and welfare of the human body. Perhaps the early Christian scholars who comprised and decided what would be included in the Bible thought the topic of bowel management too delicate a subject to include. Here is an excerpt of the translation from The Essene Gospel of Peace that Jesus shared with His followers.

'Renew yourselves and fast. Seek the fresh air of the forest and of the fields, and there in the midst of them shall you find the angel of air. Then breathe long and deeply, that the angel of air may be brought within you.

I tell you truly, the angel of air shall cast out of your body all uncleanness's which defiled it without and within.

After the angel of air, seek the angel of water. Think not that it is sufficient that the angel of water embrace you outwards only. I tell you truly, the uncleanness within is greater by much than the uncleanness without. Seek, therefore, a large trailing gourd, having a stalk the length of a man; take out its inwards and fill it with water from the river which the sun has warmed.

Hang it upon the branch of a tree, and kneel upon the ground. And suffer the end of the stalk of the trailing gourd to enter your hinder parts, that the water may flow through all your bowels. Then let the water run out from your body, that it may carry away from within it all the unclean and evil-smelling things. And you shall see with your eyes and smell with your nose all the abominations and uncleanesses which defiled the temple of your body.

Renew your baptizing with water everyday of your fast, till the day when you see that the water which flows out of you is as pure as the river's foam.

Modern day practitioners and many modern day philosophers have forgotten how destructive our diet can be to the clarity and cognition of our mind. How the quality of what we put in our stomachs affects the quality of function in our brains. They refuse or are unable to see the connection. They lack the clarity of simple stupid. Harsh but pretty on point!

The rejuvenatory powers of fasting are well documented and have been studied extensively. They have found that as we age we have a decrease in our metabolic rate, everything just starts slowing down. An experiment out of the University of Chicago placed a 40 year old man on a 14 day fast.

At the end of the 14 days his tissues were in the same physiological condition as that of a 17 year old. Yet, this is something that has been dismissed as archaic and outdated to highlight and promote the modern day breakthroughs and miracles of pharmaceutical nirvana.

Being that fasting has such a drastic effect on metabolism, it initiates the act of autolysis. Autolysis is the action of breaking down plant or animal tissue by the action of the enzymes contained within the tissue. This was recognized over 100 years ago by the medical practitioners that embraced the concept of fasting.

Fasting causes the body to digest or decompose those substances that are of least use to the body. That means that errant abscesses and tumors are promptly diminished and or completely destroyed when we abstain from solid food.

What happens is the body goes into survival mode. It will collect and distribute what is vital and very efficiently remove and destroy whatever stands in its way to survive. See, your body wants to survive at all costs, whatever it has to do it will do, you just have to supply it with whatever it is asking for or lacking.

While fasting, the body will redistribute its supply of nutrients, any surpluses and non-vital nutrients will be consumed and used first. This causes the components of a tumor, flesh, blood and bone, to be absorbed much more rapidly while the essential parts will be utilized for their nutritive value to survival.

Back to the elimination thing and how important it is for these toxins to find their way out, wherever they can. Epsom salt and baking soda baths are very beneficial in expediting the process. Even diluted hydrogen peroxide baths are very stimulating. Dry saunas are also very helpful to rid the body of toxins through the many pores in the skin.

The assimilation of food and its nutrients after a fast is quite amazing. Patients suffering from white or red blood cell deficiencies, anemia or other afflictions are typically normalized after a fast. Even dental decay is very often relieved along with loose teeth becoming fixed and bleeding gums restored.

People that were chronically unable to gain weight found that after a fast, their body returned to their ideal weight even when on a calorie restricted diet. Major deficiency diseases are also normalized due to the bodies ability to assimilate so much more effectively. It can truly be a life changer!

The body has this miraculous, built in ability to reset to near perfection or as close as will be allowed according to the overall condition and cleanliness of the whole body. Amazing seems quite weak in trying to describe the restorative power of our body and mind left to its own devices.

One of the greatest aspects of fasting is its overall total cleansing of the entire body. A systemic cleansing of not only your intestinal tract but obstructions and deposits in your lymphatic system, arteries, veins and capillaries.

Since your body is effectively cleansing all aspects and functions simultaneously, not only will the affliction you are focused on be cured or drastically reduced but other life stealing, life troubling, annoying infirmities will also disappear.

Of course the duration you choose for your fast will be determined by the severity of the affliction you are addressing and the recommendation of an experienced, alternative healthcare professional. The long standing degenerative issues will require a longer length of time on the fast.

The leading adviser and the highest rated fasting organization in the world would have to be "Fasting Center International." Anyone deciding on an extended fast of more than a week or so, I would highly recommend spending the money and contacting this organization. Especially if you are dealing with a dangerous affliction such as cancer and are taking a number of pharmaceutical medications including chemotherapy. "Fasting Center International" is widely respected and has 35+ years of fasting experience.

Extended fasts should not go unsupervised. They can be very dangerous. This company has many trained professionals that can help to guide you on a particular fast best suited to you, your goal and current medical condition. I highly recommend contacting them for support and guidance.

There is much more to fasting than just going without food and drinking water and or juice. The cleansing response can be intense. This response is not only physiological but psychological and very spiritual. Just be aware that for any extended fast it is only common sense to have the support of someone trained in the art of fasting. Trust me, your conventional doctor is not your best choice for supervising your fasting experience.

It is vitally important to start your fast in the prescribed and advised sequence of pre-fast protocols. You need to prepare for it a few days in advance. Do not decide to fill up on your favorite double cheeseburger, fries and a super big gulp, followed by a decadent slice of your favorite piece of pie and ice cream.

You need to prep your body accordingly. I know you are thinking that this fast is going to be so taxing on your comfort food addictions that you better get your fill before you dive into the deny yourself pool. Not the best approach. It may be psychologically sound according to your fear of lack and denial but not the wisest approach. This is way too serious.

The pain of watching others eat junk can be overwhelming. Try not to dwell on it. Focus on ridding yourself of whatever is ailing you. Focus on feeling and looking many years younger then before the fast and rebooting your life and your future.

...Which Water Is Best?...

The type of water you use for your fast is really important. One of the most famous and popular proponents of fasting was Paul Bragg. He along with his wife lead a fasting movement across the nation. In fact, Paul Bragg and Patricia Bragg have authored many very informative books on organic health and fasting.

They recommend using distilled water. Distilled water has no inorganic minerals in it. There are two types of chemicals, organic and inorganic. The inorganic chemicals are inert and cannot be utilized by the body.

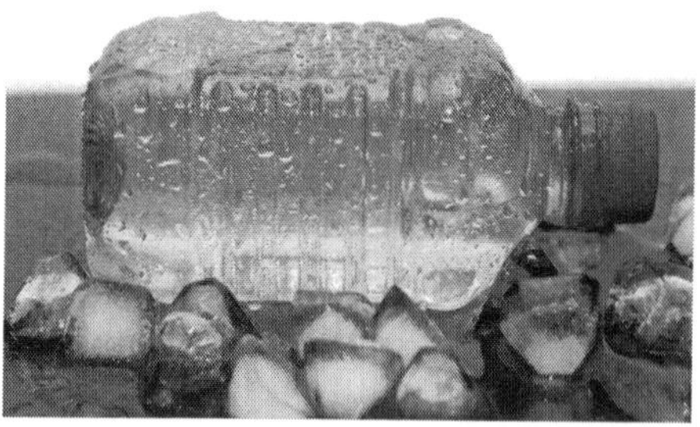

Inorganic minerals can collect on the inner walls of our veins and arteries causing hardening of the arteries, among other things. Distilled water will actually help to break down these inorganic deposits. Distilled water acts as a natural solvent. Inorganic minerals can cause a lot of problems, including kidney problems. You've heard of hard water, right? That's water with inorganic minerals in it. These inorganic minerals are very damaging to our nutritional delivery systems and can collect and impede their performance.

The distillation process removes every kind of virus, bacteria, pathogen, parasite, pesticide, herbicide, heavy metal and any other organic and inorganic material. Properly distilled water is ultra pure water. The only thing left after the distillation process is water, just plain and simple, super hydrating, beautiful, life sustaining H2O.

Everyone knows that we can only survive a few days without water, right? We have that part pretty much ingrained in our subconsciousness. It's just something we know. Probably from all the Hollywood movies depicting some poor soul struggling in the desert in a desperate search for a precious drop or two of life saving water. If he or she doesn't find water fast, the grim reaper is sure to follow.

The part I don't understand is that in our everyday life, the majority of us ignore this dire necessity. Lack of water is like the worst disease known to man. How many diseases do you know of that can kill you within a few days? We absentmindedly go through our day drinking what we think are reasonable water substitutions like; coffee, sodas, expensive energy drinks, artificially flavored teas, alcohol, pasteurized, enriched, dead, de-vitalized fruit juices and so forth. Most of us don't really give it a second thought, do you? I think we just figure any liquid will satisfy our thirst. Can you imagine what our cells think of soda pop. Don't look at me like that, you know who you are.

I think we just figure that if it's a liquid, it will satisfy our fluid requirements. Either that or we get this signal from our brain crying out for water and mistake it as a craving for food, so, off we go to the local burger joint and settle in to some cheeseburger, fry and 32oz. soda combo. Think of all the money and pounds you could have saved if you would have listened more closely. The cry was for pure, sweet, hydrating, life saving water, not a cheeseburger. Maybe you can't hear the signal anymore because the brain has just given up in frustration. It figures you never listen anyways. Just because you drink a liquid and it has water in it doesn't mean you satisfied your bodies needs. Trust me, you didn't.

Uh oh, here comes another car comparison. If only we had some of the features from our car, for instance, you can only drive your car a certain amount of miles before you need to stop for gas, yes? We need to have a mandatory stop for water? Maybe your lack of energy through the day is just that, a lack of fuel, a lack of a properly hydrated body. Maybe part of the reason your body aches and you have a hard time sleeping through the night is a lack of water. The body is so inefficient without its required fuel. Remember, your body is around 70% water, not soda, not tea, not coffee, water.

I know there is a lot of controversy over drinking distilled water and I'm sure you have heard many people say that it is dead water. You shouldn't drink it. It not only leaches minerals from the body but, a fish cannot live in it. Fish cannot live in it because they also need the natural vegetation that grows in our typical waterways and everything else that goes along with that environment. Fish couldn't live in the ocean either if it was just water. They need the entire, all inclusive ecosystem.

Part of the reason for the controversy about distilled water leaching minerals from the body is the fact that the body has to have minerals to survive. They are a part of our DNA. If the body does not receive these minerals from our foods, it will steal and leach what it needs from our bones and or our tissues. It's not the pure, free of organic and inorganic mineral, distilled water causing this phenomena. It's eating mineral deficient food. Get over it.

Water isn't water anymore with added minerals, fluoride, chlorine or other additives. Pure virgin water is H2O period, distilled water is the closet to pure H2O. The thought that distilled water leaches minerals from the body is perpetual madness. Distilled water does act like a magnet, attracting discarded and unusable minerals from the body. It then, through the assistance of the blood and lymphatic system, helps carry these inorganic, unusable minerals to the lungs and the kidneys for elimination. Distilled water will only carry away minerals that have been rejected by the cell, it in no way draws out minerals that have become part of the cell dynamic. This crazy notion is a runaway train.

Unpolluted rain water is naturally distilled and man evolved drinking collected rain water. Many ancient dwellings dating back to before Christ had reservoirs of some sort to capture distilled rain water. During ocean voyages explorers discovered native populations on tiny islands with no access to fresh water besides their innovations to capture natures perfectly distilled rainwater. Of course, nowadays, with all the pollution and smog, by the time the rain reaches the Earth it's not potable anymore.

Doctors and scientists traveled to some of these remote locations and posthumously examined some of the oldest, isolated, native people's in the world. They found an internal state of preservation they had never seen before. These people subsisted on Mother Nature's perfectly distilled rain water. Distilled water will actually help to dissolve toxic buildup in the tissue's without forming unfavorable and uncomfortable, inorganic deposits and kidney stones.

The biggest reason for drinking distilled water on your fast is that it is pure. It is chemical and mineral free. The process of distillation removes all impurities and chemicals. Although the body does need minerals it can find them much more abundantly in food. Food is our best source of bio-available, organic minerals.

Yes, food is our best source of minerals but, with the majority of our food supply grown in mineral deficient soils, supplementing is highly recommended and necessary to fulfill the bodies requirements.

Since there are no minerals in distilled water you need to take a good quality liquid, naturally balanced, trace mineral complex that includes all the essentials. It needs to be naturally balanced the way God packaged the ratios and percentages.

In fact, one of the best sources of minerals, and an absolute necessity to the body is salt. Hand processed, sun dried, millions of years old, pre-packaged and naturally balanced sea salt. Himilayan Pink Crystal Salt is the finest grade salt on the planet. It is a full-spectrum sea salt containing 84 minerals and trace minerals. Ok back to the water.

Distilled water is used to prepare liquid prescription compounds, inhalation therapies, baby formulas and it is used for intravenous feedings in hospital settings. The more I write on this subject the safer and more logical it becomes. I've done a lot of research on this subject and it always comes back to the benefits, not the detriments of using distilled water. Do not be afraid.

Most people have never been schooled on the supreme importance of hydration. It's like we have been going through life with our check engine light on. Problem is, we don't have an idiot light on our chest that reminds us to add fluids (and no, soda pop, coffee and beer are not required fluids) like we do on our car dashboard.

Did you know that most illnesses and degenerative conditions are linked to a water deficiency and imbalance? Our bodies are suffering from a major lack of water, a substantial and body dependent, water drought. Water is crucial to our health and to how well our bodies are able to perform effectively. Everything in our body is built, maintained and diluted with water. How did you possibly think you could go through life ignoring this most vital and abundant element.

When we are deficient, the body will distribute and steal whatever is available to feed certain organs, leaving other areas of the body severely dehydrated. Some areas of the body command center stage and will trump other areas of the body, especially the brain. It will not be denied its water requirements. Most of us go through life running on fumes, water vapor fumes. This isn't something that you can just brush off with the typical, oh yeah, I really need to drink more water and then add that silly little chuckle affirming the fact. It's really not funny, don't try and water down its importance. Sorry for the pun.

Of course your doctor is not going to mention how important water is to your health. They went to medical school to learn how to write prescriptions. Can you see yourself leaving the doctors office with a prescription for H2O? They don't make any money prescribing water. How stupid would that be? I can just hear the doctor now, "You know, if you would just drink enough good quality, micro-clustered, structured water, you wouldn't need to come here anymore." That's just plain bad for their bank account.

The longer we go depriving the body of water, the less we are able to recognize the bodies signals and cries for more. The intensity of our thirst perception diminishes as we grow older. Research has shown that the elderly, after 24 hours of water deprivation still have no clue or indication whatsoever of their need.

This should frighten you a bit or at least turn a light bulb on somewhere. Our blood is normally, on a good day, 94% water when properly hydrated. You need to read that again. Never mind, I'll just repeat it here, that way you have to read it again. Is that an ear full or what? Our blood is around 94% water. Sorry, I think that's mind boggling. And you thought blood was some special, incomprehensible, chemical recipe. Our blood is like water with some red food coloring added in. Our blood is truly magical, it's just that most never knew how much of our blood was water. It just screams out the point of how vital, good, clean, pure quality water is to our existence.

Ideally, our cells should be about 75% water and our brains, on average, 85% water. Energy production within the cell requires water. It provides, enables and generates electrical and magnetic energy. Inadequate amounts of water restrict the quantity and quality of energy produced within the cell. How is your energy level? Are you fatigued? Are you unmotivated? Are you lazy lately and you never used to be? Maybe your just thirsty? It's worth a shot, don't you think? It's not like you have to do a thousand push-ups or something, its drinking more water. It's fighting your way through a set of curls with a 12 oz. bottle of H2O.

...Dehydration...

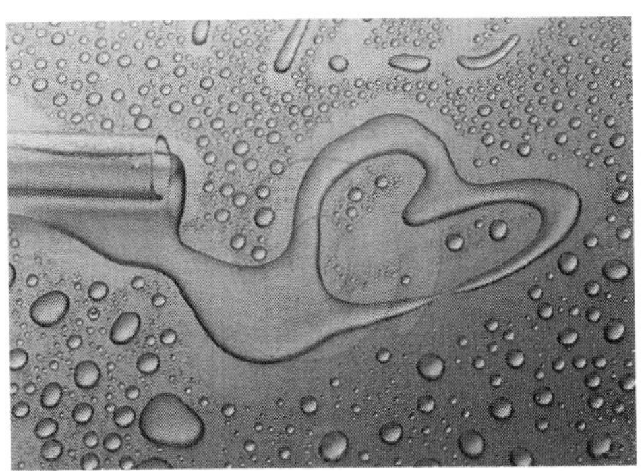

Our total and undeniable lack of water consumption leaves our bodies and our cells severely dehydrated. You would be amazed at all the mental, physical and emotional issues directly related to simple dehydration. This overly simple fix is very easily and completely avoidable. It should never have happened in the first place. Why is it not taught in kindergarten? You know what I'm saying. If water is so critical to health, why isn't it pounded into our mini minds when were the most impressionable. Kids are really smart. They remember super important things we tell them. How come we forgot to tell them?

Just think about what we go through during a drought. What happens to the vegetation, grasses and the trees? What happens to our personalities when we are continuously subjected to 98.6 degree heat with no hope of rain or some sort of moisture or cooling? That's the temperature our internal environment is subjected too, give or take a bit. What do you think happens to our cells when they are subjected to a drought condition? Never thought of it like that, did you, how long has your body been subjected to a drought? What ails you?

Most people don't even realize they are thirsty. Maybe part of the reason why you have no water impulse message being sent from your brain is because of severe dehydration. What else in your body isn't functioning properly because of this intracellular and extracellular drought?

Besides the air that we breathe, water also brings oxygen into the body. Remember that H2O thing? I know you know that O stands for oxygen. The majority of the fluids in our body are made up of water and those fluids need to be able to flow unimpeded to their destination. Those fluids are carrying life sustaining vital nutrients and oxygen. Can you pick out the problem in this picture when we don't drink enough water and these delivery systems are backed up? Those fluids need to be able to travel effortlessly to where they are needed. Major red flag when there is traffic, congestion or God forbid a pileup of plaque, yes? We have to feed our cells, they need to eat too, we have to keep them happy.

When you need to go somewhere in your car, when you need to get from point A to point B, you need to travel on some type of road or highway to get there, right? If the majority of the highways in our bodies are made up of water, how is the oxygen and the nutrition going to get to our cells without a clearly defined and free flowing, liquid highway?

You've all seen what happens to blood when someone bleeds all over the ground. Eventually the water in the blood evaporates and your left with a nasty, inert, stagnant, sticky stain. As long as the water is present it is still capable of movement, of flowing, it's still fluid and cannot become stagnant, sticky and ineffective.

Oh, I almost forgot. What do you think happens to our cells when they experience a prolonged drought? What will eventually happen to you in an extended drought? If you guessed you would die, you are really digesting the point I am trying to make. That's a good thing. I hope I am explaining it well enough for you to find the incentive to make the changes necessary to reverse your current state of decay. Believe me, we are decaying and aging beyond our numbers and years. Could it all just be a lack of water? It really could and it wouldn't hurt to try and slowly work your way up to ingesting more.

A great example of the effects of dehydration and lack of sufficient water intake is high blood pressure. This gets a lot more detailed and complicated but, keeping it simple, during dehydration, our cells build up an outer layer of cholesterol in an effort to retain whatever amount of water they have. When in dehydration mode they close up shop, they get paranoid of losing more water. They're trying to protect themselves and you.

The brain then signals to raise the pressure in your body. This is an attempt to force more water into your tissues and cells causing hypertension. Conventional doctors further compound the issue of dehydration and hypertension by prescribing diuretics. How effective could that be by prescribing something that forces more water out of the body. That's a head scratcher for me?

I understand but I still can't get my head around why they just don't tell you to drink more water. Go on a water binge. No, don't go on a water binge. You actually need to start slow and build up to the required amount.

Most alternative medical practitioners agree that your body weight divided by 2 is the ideal amount of ounces required for each day. You just need to reach that number gradually and try not to drink water during a meal. Half hour before or 2 hours after eating. We don't want to interfere with digestion if we can avoid it.

As with all the advice in this book, be sure and consult with your primary physician before attempting to increase your daily water consumption. Especially for those of you who are on prescription medications and have any heart or kidney issues. A medical practitioner skilled in hydration would be ideal. There is also a very highly recommended book by Dr. Batmanghelidj called "Your body's many cries for water." You should have a copy.

You are going to spend a lot of time in the bathroom when you initially start upping your water intake. After a few weeks your body will adjust to the increase and be able to hold on to more of the water. Also, with the increased urination you will lose a fair amount of vital minerals. Those will need to be replaced with a good liquid, trace mineral complex. You may also find that your blood pressure decreases. I'm sure your healthcare provider will be more than happy to wean you off of your prescription medications. At least they should.

There is no doubt that chronic dehydration contributes to cancer cell formation. Just think of the systems in your body that rely on and are affected by an extreme lack of water. Not only is the efficiency of the cell hindered and diminished but the removal of toxic metabolic debris and the delivery of nutrients and vital oxygen is also extremely limited. In a body that is somewhere just above 2/3 water, how can you possibly expect it to perform anywhere near healthy? It can't happen. We're denying our bodies their most crucial element. It's not lacking prescription medications and you certainly never deny it food by the ever increasing size of our waistlines. Unfortunately, water seems to always be a back seat consideration.

... Micro-clustered/Structured Water...

Now that we have been discussing the massive importance of water and what it can do to reverse many of your health issues, I wanted to give you a brief explanation of some of the newer waters on the market. When people ask me, I tell them they need to be drinking micro-clustered or structured water. They usually pretend like they didn't hear me correctly. They politely ask, "What was that?" Then I slowly repeat myself and they say, "Wait a minute, let me get a pen and a piece of paper, could you write that down please?" Just another indication of how uninformed the public is about the massive importance of hydration and the quality of the water you drink.

The majority of people think they are drinking a good quality water. Typically, your basic, mountain fed, commercially bottled spring water. You know the ones with the beautiful mountain peaks and glaciers in the background or a picture of some distant exotic beach somewhere.

If you read the fine print on the label, you'll see that it was probably bottled through some municipal water supply in downtown L.A. or something. It's all a very cleverly disguised marketing hoax. Trust me, that image you have of someone holding a container under a pristine waterfall up in the Grand Tetons is just that, an image. Now picture someone holding a container under a spigot in an industrial complex in downtown Los Angeles. That would be closer to reality for most.

Of course, I'm not saying they are bottling it straight out of the spigot. Most of them are not. At least I hope they're not. Most do filter the water or process the water to remove the majority of impurities, inorganic minerals, metals, pathogens and other chemicals. What you need to understand is that the quality control standards for bottled water are far less demanding than they are for your local city tap water. It's the big bluff, they seem so pristine and clean. The actual standards for bottled water are actually pretty lax comparatively. The biggest benefit of bottled water is that after the water is filtered it goes straight into the bottle, whereas tap water still has to travel through miles of rusty corroded, disgusting, outdated plumbing before it comes out of your home faucet.

Even if you are really drinking spring water, do you realize the amount of toxic soup and sludge we have dumped in and on our Earth? Believe it or not, that gasoline, chemical or radioactive substance that was dumped on the ground eventually makes its way into the water table and aquifers far down below. Every time it rains that toxic muck leaches further down into the Earth.

People that drink water straight from a well think they are drinking pure, nature made, virgin well water. They are usually country folks living in and around farmlands. Can you imagine the amount of pesticides, herbicides and other miscellaneous chemicals from mining and farming practices that have made their way down into the well water? I can now.

We we're country folks. We were living around a farming community and an old mining community too. We just assumed the well water was good clean, clear, uncontaminated, sparkling, fresh from the Earth well water. Right? I mean here we are in this pristine, beautiful valley with picturesque snow peaks all around us. Surely the well water was equally beautiful. My wife drank a lot of that water. Did that water contribute to her cancer? It's hard to know. The water testing company we went through said we had to be specific about what chemicals we wanted them to check for. I think it all came down to how much money we had to spend and what we could afford.

Anyway, back to the structured water deal. Micro-clustered water is water that has been broken down into smaller molecular clusters. Regular water, especially tap water, is bound in clusters of typically 10-13 molecules. Micro-clustered water is broken down into typically 5-6 molecules. The heavier, clustered, bound water configuration prohibits the water from fully permeating and penetrating the cell wall. This type of water creates a dehydration problem within the body.

Structured, ionized or alkaline water carries an electrical charge, either positive or negative. There are several different water ionizers on the market. Some of these products are quite expensive. The majority of them work by electrolysis using an anode and a cathode separated by a membrane. This process produces negatively charged, ionized water with a very absorbable and permeable hexagonal structure.

You could be drinking buckets full of bound tap water and still not be adequately hydrating your body and or your cells. Bound water also attaches to other errant molecules thereby increasing its size and impermeability even more. A lot of people find it difficult to drink large volumes of water, especially if you are going from practically no water or soda pop to half your body weight in ounces. It needs to be a slow and gradual process.

You will find that micro-clustered water assimilates and absorbs much faster into your blood, tissues and cells because of its smaller molecular size and hexagonal structure. In other words it doesn't just sit unabsorbed in your stomach like the majority of dead, de-vitalized tap waters and other commercially bottled waters. I know when I first started drinking larger amounts of water it felt like I was nursing a bowling ball in my stomach. Well structured, micro-clustered water will lessen this uncomfortable effect considerably.

Properly hydrating your body greatly enhances detox and cleansing. It will also help to reduce cellular inflammation, tissue degeneration and will help to slow down the aging process. That part just makes sense, properly hydrated skin will have more elasticity and be less susceptible to drying out, skin issues and wrinkles. The more hydrated your cells become the greater the increase and effectiveness of overall cellular function. That includes additional energy (ATP) production, and a more efficient and thorough removal of metabolic debris.

Bottom line is you need to drink copious amounts of good clean, alkaline, micro-clustered/structured water. It is required for nearly all of the therapies except for the Gerson Therapy. After reading this chapter I hope you have a greater understanding of how important and how necessary water is to our survival.

You need your body to perform like a rock star through this ordeal. Start the process immediately if you are lacking. Build up to the required amount in ounces. It will increase and multiply all bodily processes including removal of your dead and dying cancer cells.

...Fasting Con't...

If you have never fasted before it is highly advised to start with a 24-36 hour fast. You need to eat lightly for 2-3 days before you begin your fast to capture the greatest benefit from it. A variety of fresh organic salads, fresh organic vegetables, fruits and their juices. Green drinks are also recommended. Wheatgrass, barley grass, spirulina or chlorella are a few that are helpful and worthy of consideration.

Starting with a short fast will boost your confidence level for a longer, more extended fast. Also, many more people would be willing to at least try a shorter fast. Baby steps or whatever works, just keep it short and sweet and slowly build your confidence level. You can't benefit if you don't try it. You will still accomplish some cleansing on a short 24-36 hour fast.

The more practiced you get with shorter fasts, the cleaner your system will become, and the less discomfort you will feel on a longer 7-10 fast. If you are not in a hurry, than keep it to small, manageable baby steps. It's kind of like tapering off of something to make the final quit a little less stressful and uncomfortable.

The majority of us have accumulated impacted mucous and feces that is backed up in our large intestine. Since our nutrients are derived from our intestinal tract and what we have eaten, it only makes sense that a good deal of these nutrients are inadequately absorbed and toxins are getting re-circulated throughout the body and into our tissues and cells.

This chronic re-circulation of toxins, from incomplete eliminations and constipation, poisons our tissues and cells causing inflammation, an acidic environment, weight gain, water retention, irritation and dis-ease, including cancer.

Just think about it a little more in depth. Calculate about how much food you ingested during the day. Now add all that up and decide if you think what came out of you was reasonable to what you ate minus the natural absorption of nutrients. How much of what you ate that day do you think is still in there somewhere? It's just that many of us eat 3 meals a day along with some arbitrary snacking here and there and then typically eliminate only once a day. It just seems like something is getting left behind.

Have you ever noticed how unpleasant your body odor is sometimes or have you ever smelled someone's breath that smelled like feces? I have and it is totally, intoxicatingly disgusting. I was speaking to a classmate way back when and he was a close talker. I swear, without exaggerating, that a dog had just freshly done his thing in his mouth, I couldn't believe that smell was coming from his mouth. So, sorry for the visual but this is a huge indication of extreme tissue toxicity and the dire need to drop to your knees and cleanse on the spot.

Fasting is by far the most effective and quickest way to deal with massive tissue toxicity and the continual poisoning of our body and its functions.

Fasting was meant to be a regular and mandatory part of a healthy lifestyle. It is a forgotten part of our past. A conveniently forgotten part. Nobody wants to endure anything unpleasant if they make a pill that claims to make it all better, right? You know it is the sad truth and I'm no angel either.

An effective fast typically needs 7-10 days of no solid food and strictly distilled water to initiate the innate, internal healing mechanism. The goal of a fast is to reach what is called a healing crisis. This usually occurs between the 3rd and 5th day of a distilled only, water fast.

A healing crisis is when the detoxification of the blood and tissues hits a peak and some uncomfortable symptoms begin to manifest. It is when the most poisonous of toxins are dislodged and released into the body to be eliminated.

This can be a very unpleasant experience but 100% crucial to healing from any serious affliction. The poison that is trying to destroy you needs to find its way out. In the case of liver toxicity or a weakened, overburdened liver, the symptoms can be irritability, extreme tiredness, fatigue, yellowing of the skin and eyes, pain in your liver and offensive breath and body odor.

I don't want to scare you off but you have your whole life hanging in the wind and these few days of discomfort will pass, and they will have an extreme impact on the quality of your future life and health.

The best news is that this will only last a few days and the beginning of extraordinary, natural healing will have begun. The rest is up to you. You must hit this crisis, you must hit rock bottom before you bounce back and begin the journey into vibrant and enduring, radiant health. Many people decide to attempt the 40 day fast, that seems to be the magic number because it is associated with Jesus.

How much is the quality of how you feel worth? What ills and afflictions have you been managing or dealing with on a daily basis? What if they could be eradicated or drastically reduced? What if you felt 20 years younger and looked like you found the fountain of youth compared to your skeptical friends? What if, that might make it worth the trouble?

So, committing to begin with a 2-3 day cleanse is a great place to start and begin the process. Just prove to yourself that you can do this. This is going to set you up for an extended fast. Initially when you begin, the hunger hounds will be difficult to avoid but, amazingly, they ease off quite rapidly.

Just be aware of the symptoms. If you know what's coming they will not be a surprise. It's the same with anything that produces a sense of accomplishment. It does require some work, strain and stress but instead of it taking years of hard work as with your vocation, this is only days and the results from your dedication are profound.

You won't really experience too many healing reactions on a short, practice fast, except for hunger pains and maybe a slight headache. Remember this is a practice fast, something you're attempting to do to prove to yourself that you can .

I think your body actually recognizes what is happening. Your hunger pains will diminish and be quite tolerable. This is one of the reasons many are able to continue on extraordinarily long and extended fasts. After a few days the hunger pains subside considerably, let the hunger games begin. Do not be afraid, conquer your fear.

Ideally a 7-10 day fast is the average length of time it takes to more thoroughly purify and cleanse your bloodstream and your lymphatic system. The difference in how your body is able to assimilate and eliminate toxins will be nothing short of astonishing after a complete and thorough fasting protocol.

Once you get a 7-10 day fast under your belt, literally under your belt so to speak, you can contact "Fasting Center International" and commit to an extended, mind and body purifying fast of 20-40 days under superior and well experienced guidance.

Depending on the length of your fast, your intestinal tract will have contracted, so, it is important not to overeat and to be cautious of what you eat at the end of your fast. Eat something bland without spices like steamed tomato's with some garlic. You can add some olive or coconut oil for flavor and some Bragg's liquid aminos if you would like.

Always eat slowly and be sure to chew your food thoroughly to mix well with your saliva, remember, the more your food mixes with your saliva the more alkaline and the less taxing on your stomach.

Later on a fresh cut salad using cabbage, some grated carrots, beets, celery, bok choy and avocado are a good choice. You can use the juice of an orange or a lemon along with some olive oil for dressing. It would also be Ok to steam some fresh vegetables, again, making sure to chew them thoroughly and completely.

You need to re-introduce food into your system slowly. Remember if you made it through a 7-10 day fast you have initiated an incredible process of rejuvenation, recovery and enlightenment into the realms of modern day nirvana. It truly is a new beginning.

Be sure to have help, advice and guidance from a professionally trained practitioner. You also need to inform your primary physician as to what you will be attempting.

Warning: There are exclusions and warnings towards certain people that should not fast. This is a partial list of conditions and situations where fasting is not recommended:

- Anyone that is already in a severely weakened state as fasting could contribute to furthering their malnourished state.
- Fasting is not recommended for extensive carcinomas and other metastatic cancers.
- Severe liver or kidney failure
- A.I.D.S. Patients
- Children under the age of 18, as many are still developing in the growth process. Mild and short term juice fasts are Ok as long as they are properly supervised.
- Pregnant or nursing mothers.
- Advanced and extreme thyroid conditions, also people that are very advanced in age need to be carefully and preferably monitored prior to any type of fast.
- Serious heart disease, vascular disease, arteriosclerosis, post myocardial infarction, severe cardiomyopathy, Alzheimer's disease or other serious brain disorders.
- Severe manic depressives and other severe psychiatric disorders, bleeding disorders, severe anorexia or bulimia, severe anemia.
- Also people taking prescription drugs like anti-convulsion or anti-epileptic medications.

> "Fasting will bring spiritual rebirth to those of you who cleanse and purify your bodies. The light of the world will illuminate within you when you fast and purify yourself. What the eyes are for the outer world, fasts are for the inner."
>
> —Gandhi

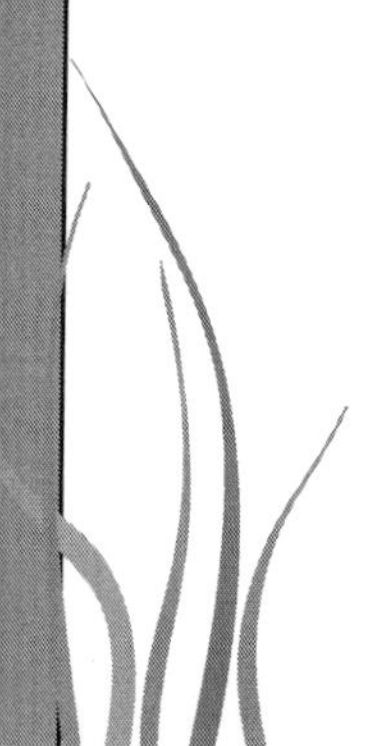

Chapter 3

Breuss Vegetable Juice Fast

This is a vegetable juice developed by a Dr. Rudolf Breuss, an Austrian Naturopathic doctor. Dr. Breuss has reportedly helped over 40,000 people cure themselves of cancer. It is a very effective juice for general detox and overall cleansing purposes also.

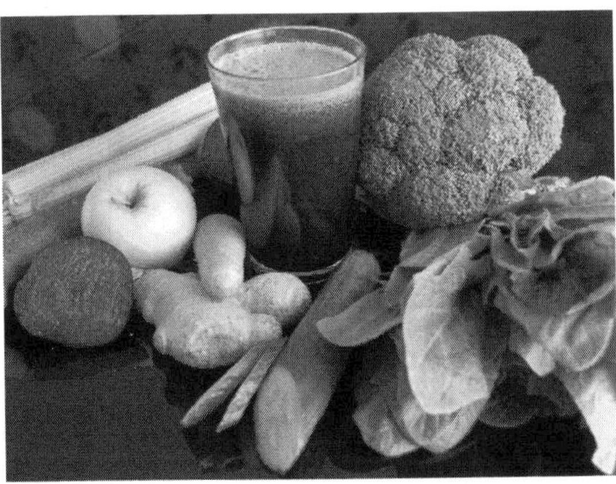

The recipe combines 10 ounces of beets, 3 ½ ounces of carrots, 3 ½ ounces of celery root, 2 ½ ounces of potatoes (especially recommended for patients with liver cancer) and 1 ounce of white turnips or Chinese radish.

This protocol relies on vegetable juices and herbal teas. The vegetables must be all organic and all sediments must be removed after juicing. Dr. Breuss also recommends drinking small amounts throughout the day. He also reminded patients to make sure to mix the juice well with your saliva before swallowing. The maximum amount of juice consumed should not exceed 500ml per day.

There are 3 different types of teas in the protocol. Kidney tea, sage tea and cranesbill tea. Dr. Breuss regarded sage tea as the most effective for detoxing the body and strengthening the immune system. He recommends drinking sage tea daily for the rest of your life.

His actual recipe calls for 2 generous cups of purified water brought to a boil in a non-aluminum pot. Lower to a simmer and add 1 teaspoon of dried organic sage. Simmer for 3 minutes and remove from the heat. Add ½ teaspoon of St. John's Wort, ½ teaspoon of peppermint. Cover and let stand for 10 minutes. Strain the tea into a container and drink 3-4 cups daily on an empty stomach.

The kidney tea is especially effective in detoxing the kidney and bladder. The kidney and bladder are extremely important as they assist the body in the removal of toxic wastes. The tea includes 3 ¾ teaspoons of the Horsetail herb, 2 ½ teaspoons of Stinging Nettle, 2 teaspoons of Knotgrass herb and 1 ½ teaspoons of St. John's Wort. Mix the herbs together thoroughly.

Preparation calls for a pinch added to a cup of purified, boiling water and allowing to steep for 10 minutes. Strain and add the dregs (leftovers) to 1 ½ cups of purified water, bring this mixture to a boil and then simmer that also for 10 minutes. Strain this mixture and then add it to the first batch. Mix together and drink ½ of a cup first thing in the morning, ½ cup before lunch and ½ cup at bedtime. Make a fresh batch each day. Discard any leftover tea.

The Breuss cancer treatment follows a very strict diet and other recommendations and restrictions. One of his restrictions was to never eat re-heated food. Dr. Breuss believed that the process of cancer cell formation relied heavily on solid food proteins. Solid food proteins are restricted except for the natural plant proteins found in the juices. One of Dr. Breuss's main theories was that cancer cells live on and inside of solid foods and if you remove solid foods from the diet, the cancerous tumors simply die off while the body continues to thrive. The fast continues for a total of 42 days.

When Dr. Breuss was in his 80's he was taken to court by the Austrian medical authority who claimed that his cancer cure was too simple and inexpensive. Dr. Breuss's attorney, himself cured by Dr. Breuss, presented a sizable group of patients cured by Breuss utilizing his Total Cancer Treatment. Surprisingly, the Austrian president also intervened on Dr. Breuss's behalf.

I only included this brief chapter and information on the juice and teas for someone wanting to incorporate these drinks into a detox regimen of their own. They would be very healing and beneficial to your efforts no matter what your affliction.

Anyone seriously interested in this protocol should definitely purchase his book (The Breuss Cancer Cure). The book will be able to more accurately guide you through the daily requirements, restrictions and foods you will need to avoid.

You can also purchase this vegetable juice from the Biotta company of Switzerland. It is a very high quality, organic juice produced with strict quality control to ensure that all vital nutrients, enzymes and other key factors are protected during processing. Many health food stores carry the Biotta brand, Breuss vegetable juice.

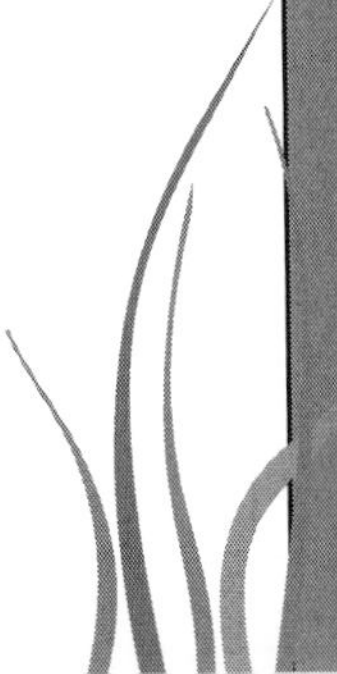

Chapter 4

Parasites

A leading scientific researcher into the cause and potential cure for cancer is a Dr. Hulda Clark, Ph.D, N.D. She describes cancer the way most other people understand it, as a fire. Once that fire has been started it cannot be stopped. This is the consensus of the majority, Dr. Clark strongly disagrees.

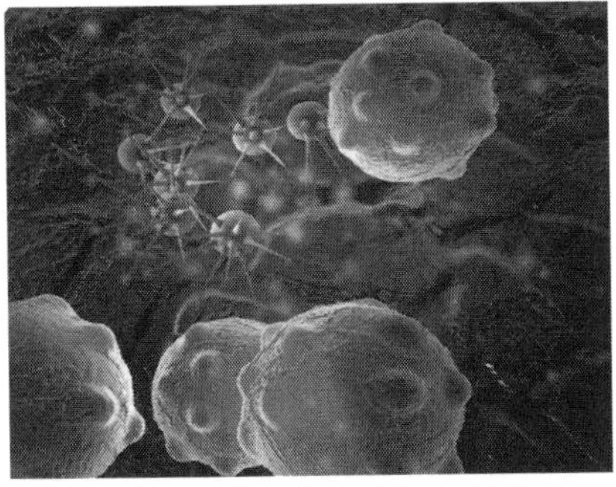

This type of reasoning has led to the process of either surgically removing the cancer if possible, intense, targeted and very destructive radiation treatments or, chemically attacking all the cells in the body with chemotherapy. This is done in the hopes of killing more cancer cells than normal cells thus, keeping the patient alive, clinging to life, with less than tolerable side effects.

The majority of the medical conglomerate believe that different cancers all have different causes. She believes this to be totally off the mark and just plain wrong. Dr. Clark believes that all cancers are alike, that they are all caused by a specific parasite. The human intestinal fluke.

She believes that if you kill and destroy this parasite the cancer will stop immediately. Sound crazy? She has some pretty convincing evidence and research to support her conclusions.

She says that the intestinal fluke typically lives in the intestines where it does little to no harm. It's when this parasite finds its way to other organs like the kidneys or the liver that cancer rears it's ugly head. In fact, Dr. Clark states that once it finds its way to the liver, cancer is the result.

She also states that in order for cancer to start and to progress, patients must have the presence of isopropyl alcohol in their livers along with the intestinal fluke.

In her book "The Cure For All Cancers" you can read about all the household products that contain some form of isopropyl alcohol. The list includes common commercial cosmetics, shampoo's, body creams, lotions, soaps, household cleaning supplies and even in our most cherished and common breakfast cereals.

We definitely live in a chemical laced, alcohol based, world of toxic soup. The majority of these items can be replaced with green, non-toxic, old fashioned alternatives. You think they were unable to clean their homes and look pretty 100 years ago? Although making and taking the initiative and effort to make the change requires discipline and commitment.

We have been deceived and brainwashed for far too long believing that harmful, fatal, and potentially cancerous products could ever possibly make it into our everyday, mainstream, personal care products. From an ethical point of view it was just assumed that health had a higher value than harm, and that this couldn't, wouldn't and shouldn't have ever happened. What happened to our value's. Seems they are being deposited into far too many greedy bank accounts.

Most people believe that parasites come from 3rd world countries where sanitation, hygiene, lack of proper food storage and sterilization, and large feral animal populations are the issue. Well, think again. It is believed that approximately 85% of the world's population of people have some form of parasitic infestation.

I know the idea of worms and parasites crawling around inside your body is a hard pill, but the statistics are valid and so are the diseases that go along with this pandemic infestation.

The more toxic you are and the more health issue's you are contending with, the greater the chance you have some sort of parasitic infestation. These little creatures can take up residence anywhere in your body. The problem being is that they steal all the nutrition that was meant for your body to use. Not only that, but after they eat, they excrete. That finds it's way into your already compromised bloodstream too.

They say that parasites can steal up to 90% of our nutrition and energy. Impacted fecal matter and a congested, mucous filled colon provide the ideal environment for parasites to flourish.

The definition of parasite is an organism that derives its food, nutrition and shelter by living in or on another organism. Unfortunately, a good majority of the time we are that organism. I know, yuck. Kind of makes your skin crawl, oops, maybe it really is.

There are over 120 different types of parasites that have been identified and over 1,000 different species. The majority being microscopic but some, like tapeworms, have been known to measure up to a foot and beyond.

These devilish creatures are able to manifest a whole host of symptoms ranging from constipation, digestive problems like gas, bloating, irritable bowel syndrome, diarrhea, muscle aches and pains, rashes, allergies, nervousness, teeth grinding, sleep disturbances, chronic fatigue syndrome, fibromyalgia, headaches, depression, obesity, sexual dysfunction, always seeming to be hungry, unexplained weight loss or weight gain and the list goes on. They can also mimic no symptoms at all, that doesn't make any sense.

Unfortunately, most conventional doctors have not been educated or trained in the diagnosis of parasitic infestations Its always something else until nothing positive is appreciatively gained by the initial diagnosis and conventional treatment plan. Hopefully, if you have an inquisitive and imaginative doctor, when nothing else is working, he then may suggest or suspect the possibility of parasites.

Sad to say that conventional medical testing procedures can typically only identify about 20-30% of infestations. Statistics show that only 30% of parasites live in the lower intestinal tract and 70% are out and about living in organs, tissues, muscles etc. This 70% of the out and about crowd of parasites are undetectable with the typical, conventional stool sample. That makes the possibility of detecting parasites outside of the intestinal tract practically nil.

A very well known author and Naturopathic doctor, Anne Louise Gittleman, ND, MS, CNS makes a great point: "If you have been suffering from symptoms you simply cannot get rid of with even the best diet, exercise, or stress relief program, chances are, parasites are the underlying cause." If you would like more information on parasites, her book: "Guess What Came To Dinner" is excellent.

Anyway, so where in the heck did you pick up a parasitic infestation? If that was your next question then food is very likely place. Especially raw meats, beef, chicken, pork, lamb and raw fish. You know how much you love that sushi/sashemi.

In the New England Journal of Medicine researchers reported finding a new parasite strain being transmitted from fish to humans. The report in the Journal describes a 24 year old student complaining of severe abdominal pain. He went into surgery to have his appendix removed. The surgeons found the appendix to be quite normal and then out crawled a 10 inch, pinkish red colored worm. The student had recently eaten sushi at a friends house, apparently, so had the worm.

Another source of parasites is water. A lot of our water is contaminated with the amoeba, giardia lamblia and cysts. Cysts are parasites clumped together. You know how polluted some of our rivers, streams and lakes are, also accidentally swallowing contaminated water during water sports or swimming is another source.

Then there's the day care center where they may not be practicing optimal hygiene, like washing their hands thoroughly after changing a dirty diaper. They can easily be transmitted and exchanged through person to person contact with an infected person.

Sexual contact, even just sharing saliva during a kiss can transmit these microscopic vermin. Remember that letting your dog or cat or whatever animal swap saliva with you is not a very sanitary practice either. I know, I love my dog too and I don't care but, I don't share his saliva anyways. Ok, anything that has to do with poop, you need to be sure and wash with anti-bacterial soap or else.

Believe it or not the fish tapeworm can reach lengths up to 30 feet+. Dr. Hulda Clark whom I spoke about at the beginning of this chapter believes that all diseases have their start with parasitic infestations and environmental toxins.

The up side to this dilemma is that through the use of some very specific herbs a great percentage of them can be eradicated. The problem with conventional treatments for parasites is that they typically only target one or two different types. The majority do not get rid of the larvae or the eggs. It's really important to hit them all and keep them from re-infesting their host, that would be you.

Unfortunately, the rate of parasitic infestations is rising. A good majority could be attributed to the rise in American's appetite for rare beef. Also, in many parts of the world sanitation practices have deteriorated. The giardia lamblia parasite is the #1 cause of waterborne diseases today.

Tapeworm infestations have increased over 100% in the last 10 years or so. Outbreaks of amoebiasis, the most feared and deadly parasitic infestation is rising too. The transmission of parasites from pigs to humans is also on the rise.

It has been reported that intestinal worms and or parasites outrank cancer as man-kinds most deadliest enemy worldwide. If you are dealing with cancer, a parasite cleanse would be highly advised. Besides cancer there are a multitude of diseases and illnesses directly related to parasite infestation. It would certainly be worth your time and effort to pursue.

The side effects of the herbal parasite cleanse is very mild in most people, it would be crazy not to address this simple yet very effective remedy. The what if's are overwhelming.

The 3 herbs in the remedy can rid you of over 100 different types of parasites. Typically without any interference from any other drugs you may be taking.

The 3 herbs in the remedy must be taken together. The 3 herbs are Black Walnut Hulls, Wormwood and Cloves. The Black Walnut Hulls and the Wormwood kill the adults and the developmental stages of over 100 different types of parasites. The cloves will kill the eggs. But again, they must be taken together.

It is critical that you purchase the Black Walnut Hulls from a reputable vendor that harvested and dried the hull while it was still green, if it turns black it is past its prime healing potential. You will need 1 ounce (30 ml) of the extra strength Black Walnut Hull tincture. You will also need 1 bottle of Wormwood capsules (between 200-300mg each) and 1 bottle of freshly ground Cloves (400-500mg each).

Once you have all the herbs listed above you can begin your treatment. The above listed amounts should last 3 weeks. If you are very ill you can speed up the protocol. The amount for a basic parasite cleanse according to Dr. Clark is as follows: Black Walnut Hull – Day one: take 1 drop in ½ cup of water. Sip it slowly on an empty stomach before a meal. Day two: Take 2 drops in ½ cup of water. Day 3: take 3 drops in ½ cup water and so on until you reach day 6 where you measure out 2 tsp in ½ cup of water.

You can mix in some fruit juice or natural sweetener to make it more palatable. If you need to progress faster you can see how well you tolerate the Black Walnut hull in the smaller doses and move up faster to the 2 tsp. a day in ½ cup of water.

Directions for Wormwood are as follows: Day 1 – take 1 capsule before dinner with a glass of water. Day 2 – take 1 capsule before dinner with a glass of water. Day 3 – take 2 capsules before dinner with a glass of water. Day 4 – take 2 capsules before dinner with a glass of water. Day 5 – take 3 capsules before dinner with a glass of water. Day 6 – take 3 capsules before dinner with a glass of water. Repeat this sequence, increasing 1 capsule every 2 days until day 14 where you should be taking 7 capsules. Take all the capsules at the same time before dinner with a glass of water. The capsules should be 200-300mg each.

After day 14, continue for 2 more days taking the 7 capsules. Then Dr. Clark recommends taking 7 capsules, once a week of Wormwood for life as a maintenance program if you are dealing with cancer. You can adjust this dosing schedule if it causes any stomach discomfort until you reach the 7 capsules.

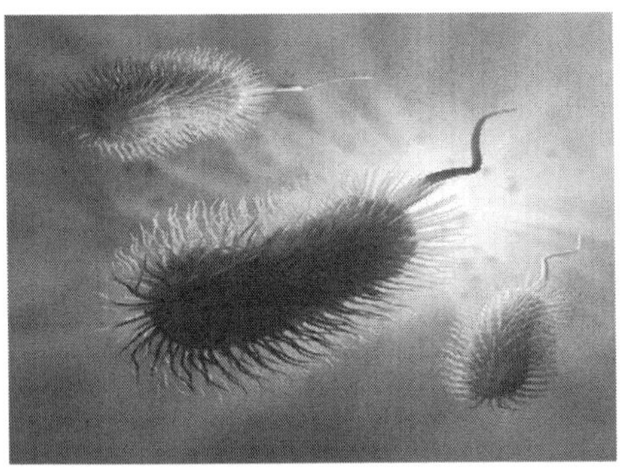

Directions for Cloves: The ground clove capsules should be 500mg each. Do not purchase your basic supermarket or herb store variety. They are typically not powerful enough and the freshness and quality is vitally important. Day 1 – take 1 capsule 3 times a day before meals. Day 2 – take 2 capsules 3 times a day before meals. Day 3, 4, 5, 6, 7, 8, 9, and 10 take 3 capsules 3 times a day before meals. After day 10, Dr. Clark recommends taking 7 capsules, all at once, once a week for life as a maintenance program.

... Parasite Zapper...

The zapper is an electronic device that creates an electronic wave called a positive offset square wave. It is set to a single frequency that creates a resonant vibration destroying parasites, viruses, fungi and other bacteria in the body.

The zapper is a device designed by Dr. Hulda Clark, Ph.D. The technology was based on the research of Dr. Royal Rife who created a resonant frequency generator that destroyed cancer cells.

To find out more about this technology please refer to the chapter in this book on the Rife Therapy. The Rife Therapy is a more than remarkable technology that had a nearly 100% cure rate against different cancers.

Dr. Clark experimented and researched the different frequencies of parasites, viruses and bacteria and developed the zapper. Being that everything in the universe vibrates at a certain frequency, targeting and creating similar frequencies or like frequencies to that particular pathogen, destroyed that pathogen.

It's similar to the wine glass that shatters when a singer reaches and resonates on a particular note. When the similar, like frequency or resonance of the glass was achieved, the glass shattered and was destroyed. This resonant vibrational frequency works in the same way. The resonant frequencies delivered by the Zapper creates this vibration destroying parasites, viruses, fungi and other bacteria in the body.

Dr. Royal Rife determined that micro-organisms all have their own very specific MOR (Mortal Oscillatory Rate). This specific rate or frequency, when amplified, will either cripple these micro-organisms from reproducing, or vibrate and destroy their membrane walls to the point of collapse, initiating the death of the micro-organism.

The Zapper produces an effect called electroporation. Electroporation temporarily increases the cells permeability. This allows medicines, herbs, vitamins and minerals to enter the cell at a greater rate and in greater quantities.

Some conventional medical doctors use EPT (electroporation therapy) to target chemotherapeutic agents more accurately. Using this technology allows the chemotherapy agent to penetrate the cancer cell membrane more effectively and reduces the actual amount needed.

Because of the electroporation effect created by the Zapper, anyone taking powerful prescription medications or powerful herbal medicines, needs to consult with their physician or other practitioner before use.

There are many different Zappers on the market and of course they all claim that their particular zapper is the best. There are dual zappers, digital zappers, frequency sweep and programmable zappers. Many of these zappers only confuse the issue and are hit and miss in their effectiveness.

If you want more information on which zapper to use you can email me and I will give you more information on the one I use. You can read up on why this particular zapper is more effective and reliable.

Chapter 5

The pH Acid/Alkaline Balance

Acidosis, (the acid/alkaline balance of your bodily fluids) and hypoxia, (not enough oxygen) are the 2 primary conditions within the body that allow germs, viruses, bacteria and cancer to breed. Changing these 2 conditions should be the first steps you take.

...What is pH anyways?...

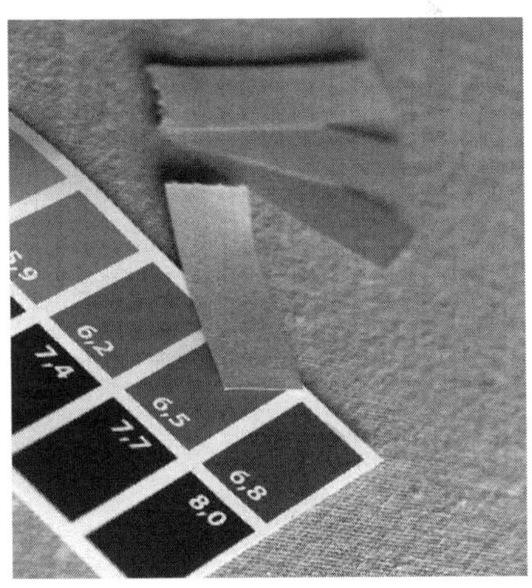

The pH is a measurement of the acidity or alkalinity, sometimes referred to as "base" of a solution. When substances dissolve in water they produce charged molecules called ions. The definition of pH is potential hydrogen. To keep it simple, even though pH is about hydrogen, the more acid a solution, the less oxygen it contains whereas the more alkaline a solution the higher degree of oxygen it contains.

Your body is constantly monitoring the pH of every body part and process. If it becomes to acidic it releases an alkaline substance to re-adjust the pH. Same thing for when it becomes too alkaline, the body releases acids to re-adjust or re-balance the pH. The pH is adjusted according to the ideal pH for that particular part of the body.

Acidic water contains extra hydrogen ions (H+) whereas basic water contains extra hydroxyl (OH-) ions and less hydrogen ions. You don't have to memorize this, Ok?

The pH is measured on a scale of 0-14. Neutral water has a pH of 7.0. Acidic water has a pH value less than 7.0, zero would be the most acidic. Likewise, basic water has values greater than 7.0, with 14 being the most basic or alkaline.

A change of 1 unit on the pH scale represents a 10 fold change in the pH, so that water with a pH of 6.0 is 10 times more acidic than water with a pH of 7.0, and water with a pH of 5.0 is 100 times more acidic than water with a pH of 7.0. Get it? Don't worry, I told you you didn't have to memorize this, Ok.

You might expect rainwater to be neutral, but it is usually somewhat acidic. As rain drops fall through our atmosphere, they dissolve gaseous carbon dioxide, creating a weak acid. Pure rainfall has a pH averaging around 5.6 and picks up a lot of pollution and smog on its way down.

Ok that's the hard part. Just understand that your body organs and fluids have different pH levels depending on their function in the body. These levels are extremely important in the battle against disease and cancer. Remember too that being overly alkaline is also dangerous.

This is a therapy that can be started immediately. It is a simple yet incredibly profound concept, in fact. Bacteria, viruses and cancer cannot survive in an alkaline, oxygen rich environment. Nobel prize winner Otto Warburg explained that there are a primary and secondary cause of disease.

He used the example of the plague, the prime cause being the plague bacillus bacteria, the secondary cause being filth, rats and the fleas that transfer this plague bacillus from rats to man.

Otto Warburg also stated that just about anything can cause cancer along with countless secondary causes. He said there is only one primary cause of cancer and that is the replacement of the respiration of oxygen in normal body cells to the fermentation of sugar in a cancerous cell.

The energy needs of our normal body cells are met by their intake and need for oxygen. Cancer cells, on the other hand, meet their energy needs in great part by fermentation. In other words, oxygen is not their friend. From a chemical and physical aspect the difference between cancer cells and normal cells could not be greater.

Oxygen is the chief donor of energy in plants, animals and humans but is completely dethroned in the cancer cell. It is replaced by the energy yielding reaction from the fermentation of sugars. During cancer cell development oxygen intake stops and fermentation begins.

So during cancer cell development oxygen is not required, in fact it is deadly to cancer cell formation. These highly different type cancer cells thrive and replicate, destroying the body and normal, oxygen rich, cellular activity.

In order to defeat this cancer the bloodstream must be kept rich in life sustaining, cancer destroying oxygen. The top scientists agree that to keep cancer away, we need to avoid as many known carcinogens as possible and keep the levels of oxygen in our cells robust and rich.

Is it really that simple? The vast majority of experts agree, and the science supports their conclusions, that cancer cannot survive in a highly alkaline, oxygen rich environment. Fortunately, we can control this acid/alkaline balance in our bodies. We can control what we put into them.

Have you noticed that just about everyone seems to be suffering from some sort of disease or imbalance? I'm sure you have, in fact, I'm sure you know of someone who is suffering from one of the big 3, heart disease, cancer or diabetes. Then again, maybe you haven't noticed.

Illness and disease are so commonplace nowadays, so accepted as a part of our reality that someone dealing with an affliction or imbalance doesn't stand out as much as they used to. It's sad, but unfortunately true, that half of us will die from heart disease or diabetes and one in three of us will die from some form of cancer.

Everyone says you have to die of something. It's almost like an accepted fact that its Ok to be ill and infirm, it's just a part of our modern way of life and our downhill decline towards death, I say, that's just wrong, that's not what God intended for us.

Most think the mapping of the human genome, cutting edge medical breakthroughs and technologies or some sort of magical pharmaceutical panacea will save us from ultimate suffering and an untimely death.

What if you didn't have to rely on the hopes of that magical pill and it was much simpler for all to achieve vibrant health and longevity? What if we didn't have to grow old with acceptable age related issues and infirmities? What if it was really simple and obtainable with something really basic, something we do everyday?.

What if all these deadly and life threatening debilities could all be controlled with diet and lifestyle changes? What if you could forget calories, cholesterol numbers, blood pressure, blood sugar and hormone levels? One of the most important measurements to protect your health is your pH, how acidic or how alkaline are your blood and your tissues?

Disease and or cancer cannot exist in an alkaline environment. The pH of our blood and other fluids regulates and affects every cell in your body. Long term over acidity corrodes body tissue and interrupts cellular activity and function, including heart beat and the neural firing of your brain. It is also what is keeping you overweight and infested with pathological micro forms.

Did you know that if you feed your body what it needs and lose the over acidic, refined, processed, preserved, enriched, artificial foods, your body would do the rest. It will re-establish your ideal cellular functions, including re-establishing your ideal weight. I know you don't believe it.

Your body is incredibly smart, remember? There is a report about a woman that was suffering from an array of different health related issues. She decided to switch from her acid/artificial diet to a healthful and well balanced, alkaline diet. She said it was the first time in her life she could actually feel her body repairing and restoring itself.

She had been contemplating surgery for her arthritis. As she progressed with her newly balanced acid/alkaline diet and life-style, her pain mysteriously diminished. She also reported that she was no longer depressed, her compulsive eating disorder vanished and she was no longer tired all the time. Her psychological and emotional relationships changed with her spouse and her children as well as her cravings for sugars and bread. One other benefit, her long time weight problem slowly disappeared.

The body is constantly trying to regulate it's acid/alkaline internal environment. Our bodies cannot endure extended acid imbalances. Early stage acid imbalances include symptoms such as allergies, headaches, skin eruptions, colds, flu and sinus problems.

If these acid conditions continue, more serious problems begin to arise including weakened organs, dysfunctional thyroid and adrenal glands, a poorly functioning liver and overall, general systemic decay. Your oxygen levels decrease from this overly acidic condition and cellular metabolism is severely interrupted.

The blood will attempt to extract alkalizing minerals out of our tissues to compensate for this imbalance. The body uses sodium, potassium, calcium and magnesium to neutralize and or detoxify a highly acidic condition in its attempt to re-regulate and alkalize.

If you eat healthy your body should have a reserve supply of these minerals on hand to meet emergency demands. If not, your body will seek out what it needs elsewhere. Calcium will be leached from your bones and teeth and magnesium from your muscle tissues. If you don't have these minerals and enzymes readily available from the foods you consume, your body will go to the mall and start shopping for it.

Remember this is a full time process your body is constantly engaged in. Your body is always working for your benefit. In other words it needs these minerals and nutrients all the time to properly manage your internal pH and internal environment. When they are not available or it has exhausted your reserves this can lead to deficiencies and other health related bumps in the road.

This continual acid load and the body constantly trying to re-balance itself, results in a vicious cycle of dumping excesses into the blood from an overfilled and or clogged up lymphatic system which in turn dumps it back into the blood.

All this is happening while the body is trying to mobilize these minerals from somewhere in the body to prevent further cellular breakdown and creating ever growing mineral deficiencies.

The fact that your symptoms are either acute, chronic or non-existent will generally indicate whether or not your body was able to locate the necessary enzymes and minerals. It needs to be able to neutralize and or eliminate these excess acids.

Your circulatory system will try and eliminate these acid wastes in liquid form through the lungs or the kidneys. When there is more than the system can handle these acid wastes get deposited in various parts of the body including the heart, the liver, the pancreas, the colon or it may deposit them in fatty tissue including: the belly, breasts, hips, thighs and the brain.

We live in a world of bacteria, viruses, fungus, mold, yeast and or other micro forms. What do they all need to ensure their survival? A low oxygen, acid filled environment and they're quite happy. Problem is, you're not!!!

When your body has to fight too long or too hard against the above mentioned micro forms it breaks down and gets noxious and overgrown with toxic pathogens. These are at the core of all that ails you.

This is part of the reason why people are overweight. Your body is actually trying to protect you by storing these acid wastes as fat and keeping them away from your vital organs.

That puts a different spin on things for you who are overweight. Part of your weight problem is your body trying desperately to protect you. Your body loves you, get over it!!!

These molds, yeasts and fungi keep your body's vital organs from performing efficiently, thereby slowing down your metabolism and energy supply. It really is a continuous and viscous cycle of internal imbalances sapping your strength and your vitality.

If you suffer from chronic indigestion or any indigestion at all, what do you do? Take a Tums? It helps for a little while sometimes but often comes right back again, right? What about listening to your body and addressing the symptom instead of looking for a way to make the symptom less obvious.

What if you addressed the underlying condition so it went away because it was repaired? Just not the way we do things here in America, sickness is a very lucrative business. We rely on the opinion of our doctors who have been trained by the pharmaceutical companies and lucky for us, they have a custom little pill to make it all better. Stop me if I'm wrong.

The digestive system is incredibly important since that is where we pick up our nutrition from the foods we eat. From there it comes in contact with our blood for distribution.

You think taking a Tums is helping to repair this massively important digestive issue? Knock knock! Stop. This is certainly not the answer, our bodies are constantly crying out for a reason, address the reason! Just flush the Tums! There's a reason why they are one of our best sellers for over the counter drugs.

Have you ever looked at what you eat in a day or 2 days. Oh my. Just for fun, try and write down every little thing you ate. I mean everything. That little piece of candy you munched, a couple of leftover chips, someone offered you a piece of chocolate, some french toast sticks for breakfast with maple syrup, a greasy, fried, fast food burger and fries with a coke for lunch and microwaved macaroni and cheese for dinner, and let's not forget that glass of milk. Holy cow, I need a Tums just writing this.

There is a constant battle going on inside of our bodies with good micro forms and bad micro forms. The good micro forms are beneficial bacteria that are supposed to be there, the bad micro forms interfere with the good. They block and displace our beneficial probiotics and hinder the absorption of vital minerals, vitamins and proteins.

When our intestinal flora (the good bacteria, the good micro forms) is unbalanced, the bad bacteria feed on the nutrients we would normally receive in a well balanced system.

The inner walls of our small intestines are covered with little projections called "villi." These villi increase the surface area for nutrients to attach themselves too.

When these nutrients latch onto the "villi,"in the small intestine, they convert them into red blood cells. These are then circulated throughout the body and converted into body cells. This sounds really important don't you think? They are constantly and continuously rebuilding our bodies.

So, keeping it simple, the quality of the food you eat determines the quality of your red blood cells, right? Which in turn determines the quality of your body cells, which determine the quality of your organs, bones, muscles etc. Ever hear you are what you eat? It's true, are you happy with what you look at in the mirror? I know, me neither.

It's really not a difficult fix. Yes you do have to give up some of your favorite foods or at least moderate them somewhat. But how hard is it to make better, well balanced alkaline food choices. I'm definitely not saying to stay away from acidic foods altogether. There is a balance to everything, just pay more attention. I'm saying stay away from processed, dead, de-vitalized, fake, faux foods. It's these acidic foods that are killing us and destroying our health.

Trouble is, we live in a world of instant results and instant, no work gratification or we can't be bothered, right? These poor eating habits end up slowly deteriorating your organs and body tissues. Part of the reason you can tell something has gone terribly awry in the way you feel.

Sad to say, it is a slow process and you typically won't feel the effects right away but, believe me, your poor food choices are slowly but surely eating away and decreasing the efficiency and quality of your vital organs. And yes, it will show up down the road. Your choice, deal with it now while there's time or deal with it when it comes and threatens your life. Trust me, it will come.

Why are we so stubborn? I hear people say I'll deal with the problem when and if it appears. I love my so and so and I will not give it up for all the tea in England, ha, you thought I was going to say China. So why do we do this? So many foods are our drugs. If you were thinking you were not a drug addict, you really are. It's just that your drug has been very cleverly concealed in a food item that you can't live without. Think about it. What's the difference?.

Eating these toxic foods and relying on them for our nutrition is like constructing a building with inferior blocks, the building will go up just fine. It will stand and yes you can even live in it. Problem is the blocks are inferior so, they will eventually fail and they are slowly breaking down and disintegrating. But who cares, right?

Everything is fine right now, it looks Ok. Hang onto that instant gratification and instant result. Enjoy your new home while it is still standing. Just remember when the building comes tumbling down somewhere down the road, you knew it would happen, you built it. Trouble is, you are going to be in it when it fails!

Same thing with your body. You are building it with the foods you eat and the liquids you consume. Are you going to want to live in it in 20 years, 30 years? It's still standing. I bet you won't. It's coming, you know. Are you using inferior materials? Your digestion is extremely important. You probably already know if yours is functioning well or not, don't you?

Too many people think that taking some live culture probiotic will fill the bill and take care of the problem. Not true, yes it is very beneficial but, you have to make dietary changes too. If you don't the little fellows will just pass straight on through. You have to keep a clean house to entice them to stay.

I'm sure many of you have tried this technique with little benefit, right? Once again it is the internal environment that determines whether or not they decide to hang out. Keep them happy, they are your BFF's.

I know you hate to hear this but raw and lightly cooked fruits & vegetables are your best line of defense. They are the most nutrient dense foods on the planet. They provide all the minerals, vitamins, proteins and micro nutrients your body needs to function at its best. Besides the vitamins and minerals, they also provide chlorophyll, soluble and insoluble fiber, enzymes, phytonutrients and crucial, alkaline, natural salts. Yes your body has to have salt, it just has to be the right kind of salt. And no, that salt in your canned corn is not the right kind of salt.

Nature has provided us with an excellent cleanser found in fruits and vegetables. It's called fiber, ever hear of it? And no, animal products contain absolutely zero fiber. Fiber has been shown to drastically decrease mycotoxicity. It acts like a sponge soaking up excess acids from the body. Fiber also acts like a broom, sweeping and cleaning out our intestinal tract.

Enzymes are the foot soldiers used by our bodies for just about every chemical activity and function in the body. We need boundless supplies and reserves of enzymes.

Unfortunately cooking your food above 120-130 degrees destroys enzymes. This is why it is so important to eat as much raw, uncooked, organic fruits and vegetables as possible. When we exhaust our enzyme supply, our front line of defense, the Marines of the body, we die!

Another critical aspect of your diet, although it is not specifically food, is to thoroughly chew your food. I don't want to sound like your Mother, but, there is an old saying, "drink your solids and chew your liquids."

I know it sounds crazy but the body and all of its intended parts really do partake in a carefully executed chorus of synchronicity. Stop inhaling your food like it was vapor, stop with the "Get er done" style of mastication, try actually enjoying your food and the experience.

I'm sure I've said this already in this book, either that or this is the first time and I'll end up saying it again later, but, don't you see the benefit of chewing your food? Try and visualize. Your body is very busy, when you eat like a wolf, you tie up some vital resources that could be doing something really important for your health. Give your digestion a break, don't swallow that mouthful just yet!

That means chewing solid food until it is almost a liquid. This obviously helps lessen the amount of digestion necessary to extract the nutrients and it also alkalizes the food with the combination of your saliva.

That is part of the reason why they say to chew your liquids. Your saliva helps to alkalize anything you put in your mouth. Indigestion? Try chewing your food more thoroughly. Also, eating slower and chewing your food will actually satisfy your hunger sooner and you won't feel the need to eat as much. Research confirms the fact that eating till nearly bursting is very unhealthy. Everybody wins when you chew.

When you rush through a meal you never give your stomach a chance to register it has had enough. This is all very important in your battle against disease and changing your body's pH.

The bottom line on your pH is that it affects the quality and functionality of all your body processes. Your body was designed to naturally destroy foreign, harmful, pathogenic and carcinogenic substances.

It has been weakened by our highly acidic, refined, overly processed western diet. Look up the food chart of acid/alkaline foods. Make a copy, refer to it prior to every meal, it's really pretty simple.

Your plate should consistently be around 80% alkaline foods and 20% acid. Our modern diets are typically the other way around. 80% acid and 20% alkaline.

You need to eat more alkaline, oxygen rich foods. Eat as much raw, organic, alkaline foods as is reasonable. As close to 80% raw as possible. Purchase pH test strips and keep track of your levels diligently and daily. They are not 100% accurate but will give you a general indication of where your at, at least for your urine and saliva. Just read and follow the directions.

It is a very delicate balance. You should also try and eat a portion of your foods lightly cooked or steamed, it will help with digestion.

Drink pure, alkaline, micro-clustered water. About 6-8oz glasses daily. Drastically reduce your consumption of high acid foods, mainly animal products, by-products and dairy, they are all highly acidic.

Too many people believe that some newly marketed, state of the art health supplement holds the answer to their less than ideal state of health. That overly marketed, supreme, multivitamin. It's not going to happen, quit wasting your money. Whole fruits and whole vegetables in a capsule is your best bet. Otherwise make it happen in your food choices.

Your only making someone else's bank account healthy with their ridiculous claims about their supplement. And yes, they are going to make you promises ripe with emotion to profit from your guilt and or your fear. Our vitamins and minerals need to come from our food in whole, specially balanced amounts and percentages.

They are simple, easy to understand, straight up necessities for good health. There is no magic pill or supplement that will save you from your bad decisions of what you put in your mouth. Now that you are sick or infirm in some way, now it has your attention.

You will need above all else, good, clean, sweet, salt of the Earth, oxygen. Find it wherever you can. You will also need water, minerals, vitamins, enzymes, a sparkling clean colon, the natural energies of the Earth and good old mental, emotional and spiritual balance.

...All About Minerals...

Oxygen is the greatest detoxifier and organ/tissue cleanser on the planet. Thing is, bugs, parasites, bacteria, viruses and other toxins hate oxygen, it is not their friend. You also need a good whole based complex, liquid trace mineral complex daily. Minerals are the catalysts for the chemical reactions that take place between the cells in the body every second.

Minerals maintain the alkaline balance of the blood and the skin and help carry oxygen's electrons around the body. In fact a lack of minerals in your body prevents vitamins from doing their work effectively.

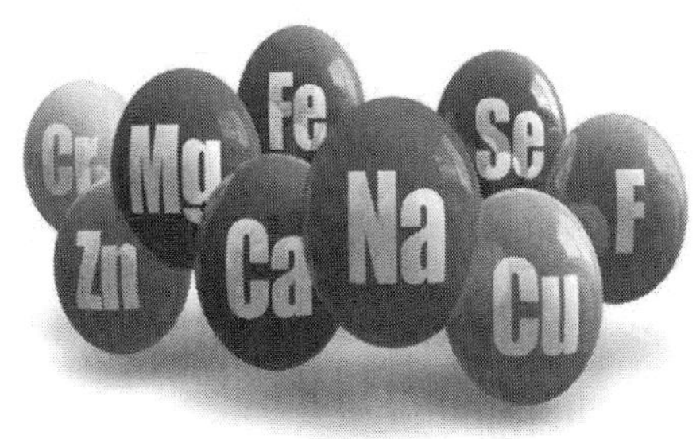

Minerals maintain the inter-cellular communication channel functions. They are crucial. How long have you been taking some isolated vitamin supplement and noticed that nothing has really changed. Vitamins have to have minerals, if you don't have the required minerals to activate and utilize the vitamins you might as well save your money. Your seriously not helping yourself.

We eat our food, chew it down thoroughly (hopefully) and it arrives in the stomach where, along with enzymes, it is broken down by digestive acids. Our bodies literally break down the foods into their isolated component parts, you know, what they were before they were assembled by Nature and the soil and turned into something we could wrap our lips around.

The purpose of eating is to distribute and absorb these minerals into our bodies where they are absolutely necessary for our bodies to function, heal, rebuild and repair.

Minerals are one of nature's greatest tools. Pharmaceuticals on the other hand have no minerals, they have no purpose or need in the body. They leave the problem firmly in place and cover up the bodies messaging system. Drugs are the lazy man's route, thing is, they are the route to further deficiencies.

The mineral content of our soils is dust, literally dust, the majority of them are gone, depleted! Your body was built on minerals, it has to have ALL the minerals to repair itself. Not surprisingly they actually change the taste of the food.

We have all sorted through the carrot bag hoping we luckily score one that is sweetish and palatable. You know what I'm talking about?.

Ever notice how some of them are bitter and disgusting. The reason for this is the carrot was grown with only production in mind. The carrot was harvested before its time in mineral less soil, and never had a chance to absorb whatever minerals may have been present. Its natural sugar state was denied by the early harvest. There's a reason the word "ripe" is in the dictionary.

They tested the mineral content of a typical salad today and found that you would have to eat a salad the size of a bathtub to obtain the same mineral value of a basic salad 60 years ago. It took 75 servings of spinach to equal the amount of iron in a single serving of spinach 50 years ago.

A great example of the necessity for minerals would be calcium and oxygen. They are crucial components of our bodies function. They help to absorb lactic and carbolic acids from our metabolic activity. Legitimate coral calcium, similar to the brand I personally use is from Okinawa and contains 75 trace minerals. Minerals are vital to oxygen transport.

These are amazing components from the sea that are millions of years old and contain all the essential minerals necessary to sustain life, a healthy and healing life.

I'm sure you have heard people claim that you shouldn't take this or that mineral with this mineral or this mineral with that vitamin, right? That's because they have been isolated and fabricated by man, assigned a milligram amount and then an educated guess of its RDA (recommended daily allowance). I'm going to trust God's RDA.

These minerals are crucial to balance your body pH. And yes, you need to take them all together. Together the way nature balanced them, as a complete complex. Precisely measured amounts in their natural, unadulterated, whole form or condition. Stay away from vitamins that are taken apart or extracted in a lab somewhere.

The acid/alkaline level of your blood is of prime importance and minerals play a crucial role. Your heart pumps over 100 quarts of blood per hour. Acid based blood can do serious damage to the heart tissue and muscle. Then there's your hearts critical need for oxygen rich blood, just thought I'd mention that.

Remember that what you decide to put in your mouth effects the pH and oxygen content of your blood. Remember too that everything in your body is all tied together. Everything has to have oxygen rich blood, vital minerals and essential vitamins! Feed it or deny it. I could go on about your other organs but I think you get the picture. You know how important oxygen rich, alkaline blood is to proper immune system function.

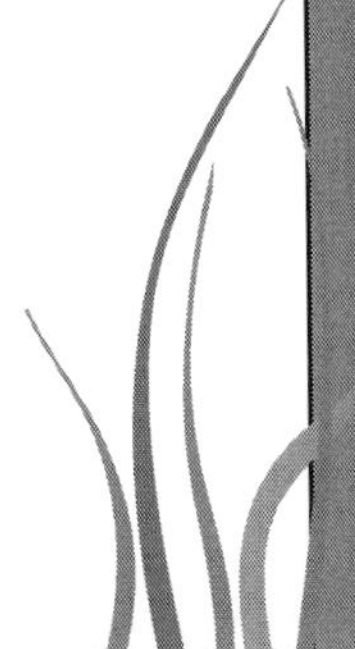

Chapter 6

Essiac Tea Remedy

"Clinically, on patients suffering from pathologically proven cancer, (Essiac) reduces pain and causes a recession in the growth; patients have gained weight and shown an improvement in their general health. Remarkably beneficial results were obtained even on those cases at the "end of the road" where it proved to prolong life and the quality of life. The doctors do not say that Essiac is a cure, but they do not say it is of no benefit."

—Dr. Brusch & Dr. Charles McClure.

"For I have in fact cured my own cancer, the original site of which was the lower bowels, through Essiac alone."

—Dr. Charles Brusch, M.D.

This remedy came about through a Canadian nurse named Renee Caisse. She obtained information about the formula through a patient in the hospital where she worked. This patient had cured their own cancer using the tea.

The story is that she received this tea recipe from an Ojibway Indian herbalist. There is some debate as to where the recipe came from, nonetheless, its efficacy stands firm through many eyewitness accounts of its healing ability.

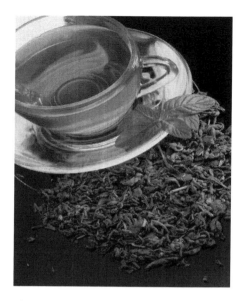

Renee Caisse moved to Bracebridge, Ontario, Canada in 1922 and began administering Essiac tea to all able and willing participants. For the most part, these were patients that had been given a terminal diagnosis from their physicians and given up with no hope by the conventional medical authority.

Renee Caisse obtained and prepared the herbs and tea at her home. She then began administering the tea orally and by injection. Patients with severe damage to vital organs, either from the cancer or from the use of conventional therapies (chemo), still died, but, they lived much longer than expected and many of them passed in considerably less pain. Others considered terminal and without damage to vital organs were cured by the tea and lived 35-45 years after their original diagnosis.

Unfortunately Renee Caisse met with extreme prejudice from the Canadian Ministry of Health and Welfare and the Parliament. A petition was signed by friends, former patients and family members to try and legalize her right to administer Essiac Tea freely and without interference.

Sad to say, it was denied. She was continually harassed by Canadian authorities. The only reason she was not imprisoned was because of support from the town council in Bracebridge. She also had the support of many well known doctors and obviously her many patients that were recovered and or cured.

Renee Caisse was forced to treat only terminally ill patients. In order for Rene to continue administering the tea she had to secure the credentials of an established and licensed medical doctor for diagnosis and prognosis. She was also told she could not accept any monies for her services.

She agreed to the conditions and stated "I never dreamed of the opposition and the persecution that would be my lot in trying to help suffering humanity with no thought of personal gain".

The treatment with Essiac Tea was not something that was shouted across the media and into the public domain. It was a dark horse in the well lit arena of deceptive bureaucracy.

Seems the tea could seriously hamper the burgeoning and highly profitable chemotherapy industry. So the powers that be, the ones who realistically make the decisions in this world, kept a very close guard on any public exposure of the Tea.

In 1977, a year before she died, she made a deal with what she thought was a large pharmaceutical subsidiary (Resperin). She figured they had the power and funding to get Essiac Tea out into the hands of the suffering public. So she offered them the recipe and formula for the tea.

Unfortunately, this company seemed to be breaking bread with the Canadian authorities and her dream of worldwide exposure on the effects of Essiac Tea disappeared into obscurity.

Sometime later a California chiropractor named Dr. Gary Glum had heard about the healing properties of Essiac tea and set into motion his own search for the original recipe and formula.

Dr. Glum finally stumbled onto the original formula from someone who had been cured with the Tea. He ended up buying the formula from this person after confirming its authenticity. Dr. Glum also obtained further information about Renee Caisse from a Mary McPhearson. It turns out Mary was a close personal friend and also a patient of Renee's, she had also started working with Renee back in the 1930's.

Dr. Glum began writing his book "Calling of an Angel" which told the story of Renee Caisse and her amazing successes treating cancer with the formula. In his book, Dr. Glum openly offered how and where to obtain the recipe for the tea.

Sadly, Dr. Glum was forced to self publish his book because of its threat to the incredibly lucrative cancer industry. Doesn't that make you sick to your stomach to attach the word industry to such a horrific disease, as if it was some worthy stock and blossoming start up investors should take a serious look at.

There was also the potential for wrongful death lawsuits against any publishers since the tea was not approved by the FDA. Dr. Glum was continually harassed by U.S. Marshals and nearly completely ruined financially through false claims by the IRS.

It was also mentioned that Dr. Glum was confronted by a naval intelligence operative who threatened his life and the life of his family members if he continued to publish his books, "Calling of an Angel" and "Full Disclosure" Full disclosure reveals details about the controversial birth of the AIDS virus. A very interesting read if you are somehow able to track down a copy.

He remained in harms way for sometime. There are very few of his books still available but, there are summarized versions still available online in PDF format but, who knows, it may have disappeared beyond recovery. Worth the time if your so inclined.

With Dr. Glum's strong belief in the tea, he got involved with AIDS Project Los Angeles. They had, at the time, 179 terminal AIDS patients. Their weights were down to about 100lbs and their T-cell counts were below 10. They were very close to death.

The Project agreed to give Dr. Glum 5 of these patients. He took them off of AZT and DDI and changed them over to the Essiac Tea 3 times a day. Incredibly, those are the ones who survived, the other 174 died.

This information is also not readily available to the public since AIDS is another blossoming moneymaking industry.

Dr. Glum shared the story of a young boy he treated with the Tea who had terminal leukemia. The young boy made a complete recovery only to die later on from heart failure. An autopsy later determined that the chemotherapy treatments had caused his heart failure.

During Dr. Glum's research regarding the tea, he met a Dr. Charles Brusch who ran a cancer clinic in Boston. He was the personal physician for the late John F. Kennedy. Turns out Renee Caisse worked with Dr. Brusch at his clinic between 1959 and 1962.

Dr. Brusch successfully treated his own cancer and the cancer of Ted Kennedy's son, who had an incurable form of cancer with the tea. After treatments with the tea they surprisingly found no trace of cancer left in his body. Soon thereafter, Dr. Brusch was hit with a gag order and told to keep his findings to himself or end up in a military prison for the rest of his life. Certainly not the response you would think.

Dr. Glum shares a quote in his book from Dr. Brusch that states "The results we obtained with thousands of patients of various races, sexes and ages, with all types of cancer, definitely prove Essiac to be a cure for cancer. All studies done in four laboratories in the U.S. and one more in Canada fortify and validate this claim."

Within days of Renee Caisse's death, authorities ransacked her house and burned all of her records. Fortunately, her friend and associate, Mary McPhearson had saved a few of Rene's records and through a series of autobiographical articles those records became public.

Dr. Glum stated that the reason the information on Essiac is withheld is because cancer is the second largest revenue producing business in the world next to the petrochemical business. The moneymaking power brokers protect themselves by suppressing and burying the truth. He explains that no one has ever actually sought out a cure for cancer, only to control it.

All the research institutes, the federal government, the pharmaceutical companies and anybody else that has stock in the massive healthcare of cancer, including our largest charities like the American Cancer Society, the Canadian Cancer Society and all the others that claim to raise money for the cure are all intricately involved in the money and power around cancer. They all have significant influence over regulatory agencies like the FDA, AMA etc.

So much effort put forth by so many trusting souls to organize and advertise massive fund raising events. They firmly believe these organizations of science are seeking that all elusive cure. It is elusive for a reason. You can fill in the rest of this paragraph.

Alternative treatments are not legal, the only legal practice and treatment for cancer is through surgery, chemotherapy or radiation. Anyone practicing otherwise has sadly been shut down and forced to move elsewhere, like another country.

It has been determined that Sheep Sorrel is the herb responsible for killing cancer cells. This information was passed on by a Dr. Chester Stock at Memorial Sloan Kettering in New York to the Canadian Ministry of Health and Welfare. It was immediately banned for sale or distribution by the Canadian government. It sadly seems the song remains the same.

Dr. Glum even went to 60 Minutes producer Philip Scheffler. He had read the book by Dr. Glum "Calling of an Angel" and was asked by Dr. Glum what he was going to do about it. No response. Dr. Glum reiterated that all the information in the book was true, Dr. Glum said, you're 60 Minutes, why don't you expose me and the tea as a fraud?

Dr. Glum then took it to Joe Donally, producer for ABC in New York. Dr. Glum said "why not give it to Peter Jennings, Geraldo Rivera, Ted Koppel, one of those?" He said they couldn't do it because they would be flooded with phone calls, besides the fact he was looking forward to retirement and had a mortgage.

Seems nobody wants to step on the toes of the power elite that pay their salaries and advertise with their networks. The cancer business is far too big and way too powerful even for the largest media sources that are esteemed to tell us the truths nobody else will.

Bogus reports were even issued stating that the tea had no beneficial results whatsoever, even when a man listed in their reports as being dead, showed up at Renee Caisse's door and thanked her for the blessing of Essiac Tea.

In Renee Caisse's own words, she said, "if Essiac doesn't have any merit it will kill itself." Amazingly it has survived all these years simply by word of mouth. As long as people had the correct recipe and the correct herbs it would stand on its own.

Renee found also that Essiac Tea would help to normalize the thyroid gland, heal stomach ulcers within three or four weeks and she had clinical cases where patients on insulin discontinued it by using the tea.

Dr. Glum also reported that he has been in perfect health since starting on the tea, no colds, no flu, he sleeps well and has noticed an increase in energy. Part of the beauty of natural therapies is the effect on other existing afflictions, they too will respond to changes.

Remember there are unethical practitioners in every arena. Alternative medicine is no different. The same deceptive practices are common across the board. It's not just conventional, allopathic medicine encouraging return visits and multiple applications or treatments.

Repeat clientele pays the bills every month. No one wants to find a cure for cancer or AIDS, remember, it is the second largest money making medical monster in the world next to the petrochemical conglomerate.

There are many different versions of the tea available, all claiming to be the original Essiac formula. The original formula contains Burdock Root, Sheep Sorrel, Slippery Elm Bark and Turkey Rhubarb in their proper ratio's. The quality of the herbs is also extremely important.

Many are using irradiated herbs since many of the herbs are purchased and grown overseas. Try and find herbs grown here in North America if possible. They should all be verified and certified organic.

Sheep Sorrel is an anti-cancer agent and is being used effectively to break down and reduce tumor tissue. The rutins and polysaccharides in Sheep Sorrel help to prevent and dissuade cancerous growths. Sheep Sorrel is also rich in beta carotene which helps to increase the production of cancer killing T-cells.

Sheep Sorrel along with the Burdock Root helps to cleanse the bloodstream. Sheep Sorrel is also being used to reduce the side effects of chemotherapy. Sheep Sorrel can be used as a topical wash for skin conditions including poison ivy, rashes, herpes, eczema , insect bites and other skin afflictions. Sheep Sorrel made into a poultice can be used on cancerous tumors for its drawing affect.

Every part of the Sheep Sorrel plant is used medicinally. The chlorophyll in Sheep Sorrel has many amazing benefits. It helps to decrease swelling, promotes tissue regeneration, strengthens cell walls and assists the liver in detoxification. Many herbalists recommend Sheep Sorrel for digestive problems, infections, cold sores, hemorrhoids, fevers and scurvy. It is also used to treat kidney and urinary disorders.

Burdock Root is one of the best blood cleansers known. It has great benefits to the skin, helps to sooth the kidneys and helps to break up congestion in the lymphatic system. It increases urine production and is helpful in weight loss. It is also very effective against skin irritations and other skin abnormalities. It has anti-inflammatory properties, helps rheumatic conditions, pulmonary affections, gonorrhea, gout, sciatica, syphilis, pimples, boils, colds, fevers and other immune system disorders.

Slippery Elm Bark has many medicinal applications. It is used internally as a mucilaginous herb to soothe and coat inflamed mucous membranes. It is very soothing for digestive disturbances including duodenal ulcers, irritable bowel syndrome, hemorrhoids, gastritis, colitis and heartburn.

It effectively draws out impurities, disperses inflammation and speeds up the healing process. Although it is rather bland it is an excellent sustaining food especially for weaning babies and the elderly as it is very gentle on the system. It contains as much nutrition as oatmeal. It is one of the few that can be tolerated when nothing else will. It is extremely easy to assimilate and eliminate even for very delicate stomachs. It will absorb noxious gases and help to neutralize an acid stomach.

Because of its soothing properties it is also used externally for skin eruptions, burns, poison ivy, boils, abscesses, vaginal irritations, tumors, chapped skin and other skin afflictions.

Turkey Rhubarb helps to promote the actions of the liver and flow of bile. It also helps to increase saliva and the flow of gastric juices. It stimulates the muscular layer of the bowel increasing peristalsis (peristalsis is the contraction and relaxation in the muscle of the large intestine which helps push what our body didn't use towards its exit point). It is only used in small amounts as it will help to alleviate a stopped up bowel. It is very often used as a laxative for its stimulating effects.

Turkey Rhubarb will help to remove any irritating substance in the bowel that may be causing diarrhea. It is frequently used as a laxative for children and infants because of the milk like quality of its actions. It just needs to be administered by someone knowledgeable in its application.

For the tea, the Burdock Root should be cut and sifted, the Sheep Sorrel needs to contain the roots for optimal efficacy and brewed in its powdered form. The Slippery Elm Bark and the Turkey Rhubarb should also be powdered. Make sure to purchase and use Turkey Rhubarb Root and not Rhubarb Root. Just keeping it real.

You can purchase the tea already bottled at most health food stores but I think you are much safer brewing it yourself or having a local herbalist brew and bottle it for you. I just don't trust the quality and effectiveness of the mass produced tea. I like to know what goes into it, and certainly know there are no additives or preservatives. It needs to be as fresh and pure as the Earth itself.

The best place to find out more information on Essiac Tea and to purchase the proper ingredients including the Sheep Sorrel with the roots is through http://healthfreedom.info.

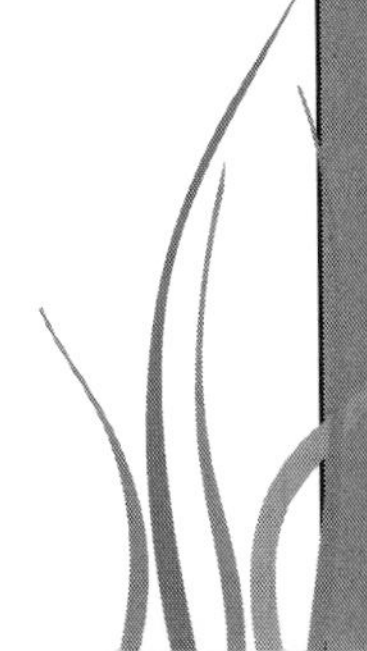

Chapter 7

Ozone/Oxygen Therapy

Number 1, everyone of our cells has an absolute requirement for oxygen. Cancer cells on the other hand thrive without oxygen. Oxygen is what gives your blood its bright red color, the darker the color of your blood the less oxygen it carries whereas the brighter the color the more oxygen saturated it is.

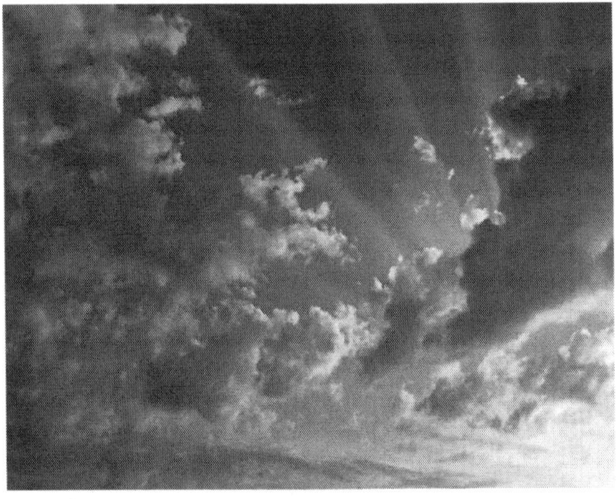

Freshly oxygenated arterial blood is delivered throughout our body to our cells and then returned to the lungs for re-oxygenation.

This is one of the reasons why blocked arteries or narrowing of the arteries is so harmful to the body. When the oxygen carrying arterial blood is impaired or hindered in any way, so is the delivery of oxygen to our cells. This can initiate disease and cancer cell formation.

Oxygen seems so simple, too simple. I mean sure we need it to sustain our life, we have to breathe, but how incredibly vital and how deeply does the overall need and necessity for this invisible gas go?.

...What Is Ozone Anyway...

You know about the Ozone layer above the Earth. That layer that protects us from the damaging effects of ultraviolet radiation, right?

A lot of people have been told that Ozone is smog. That is actually very far from the truth, even so, some will still try and convince you otherwise. Ozone is actually an energized form of oxygen with extra electrons. The majority of smog on the other hand is really hydrocarbon based particles. Thick, black, sooty, lung choking hydrocarbons, Ozone is a colorless gas, a big difference.

Ozone is measured in parts per million so it is microscopically small in size. The reason it is associated with and a part of smog is because it is negatively charged. That is a good thing. It is one of our most efficient and effective anti-oxidants and air purifiers. Truly a gift created by God.

Anti-oxidants scavenge and attract positively charged free radicals, but you already knew that. Free radicals are compounds with unpaired electrons looking for something to bond with.

...Where Does Ozone Come From?...

Ozone is produced naturally. Ozone is created when oxygen molecules are broken apart by the sun's ultraviolet energy into single oxygen molecules (O1) in our upper atmosphere. Since oxygen, O2, consists of 2 oxygen molecules, when 3 oxygen (O2) molecules break apart, they produce 6 singlet oxygen molecules. These 6 singlet oxygen molecules quickly recombine into two O3's, 3 oxygen molecules bound together create an ozone molecule.

In fact these singlet oxygen molecules can now recombine into longer chains of ozone molecules. When 3 or more oxygen molecules bind together, they create O3, O4, O5, O6, O7 and so on. Ozone molecules are so energized and unstable that they are constantly looking to become stable oxygen molecules again. They do this by giving up their extra, singlet oxygen molecule. This is how ozone begins its healing reaction. These negatively charged, singlet oxygen molecules begin scavenging for the positively charged free radicals in our body. They then attach to these free radicals and oxidize them.

This is a constant and consistently happening phenomena. As long as the sun is shining, ozone is being produced. Ozone then falls toward the Earth, being that ozone is heavier than air. Another benefit of ozone is that as it falls to Earth and passes through moisture or clouds it gives up singlet oxygen molecules which quickly recombine with the moisture or water, H2O, and form H2O2, hydrogen peroxide.

This trace amount of H2O2 along with H2O then continues falling to the Earth in rainwater. The roots of plants and trees then take up this extra oxygen rich water. This oxygen rich rainwater also makes its way into our aquifers. We draw drinking water from the wells and eat the fruits, vegetables and grasses which are much more vibrant and nutritious now depending on the amount of oxygen rich water absorbed from the soil.

Cascading waterfalls and waves crashing on the sand lessen the surface tension between water molecules and stretch their surface area allowing room for extra singlet oxygen molecules from the air. Ever notice how refreshed and energized you feel after spending time in the surf, downstream from or under a waterfall? This is from the exchange of singlet oxygen molecules. Simple, right?.

I'm sure you have noticed how much faster your grass seems to grow and how much greener and more vibrant it seems after being watered from a fresh rain shower compared to watering it with the dead water coming from your local garden hose. This is the natural circle and cycle of life in this giant biosphere we live in called Earth. It is a constant and continuous cycle. Anywhere there are extra singlet oxygen molecules; toxins, microbes and pollutants are being devoured and denied their right to life.

...How Does The Ozone Layer Protect Us?...

The ozone layer protects us by using the sun's damaging but energized ultra violet rays to break apart O2 (oxygen) into singlet oxygen molecules in our upper atmosphere. The higher the oxygen content of our air from plants, trees and other vegetation, the greater the amount of ozone created. The greater the amount of ozone created, the greater the amount of the sun's harmful UV rays are depleted creating this crucial reaction. So simple, so precise.

This is the truth behind the destruction of the ozone layer. The more polluted our air becomes, the more our oceans are used as a toilet for anything and everything, and the more oxygen producing vegetation cut down and destroyed, the less oxygen available to create ozone and reduce the sun's damaging ultraviolet radiation. We desperately need as much available, salt of the Earth oxygen as possible to oxidize and eradicate the enemies of dynamic health.

Oxygen is the king and free radicals, toxins, microbes and other pollutants are mere paupers in its presence.

You know the story about how opposites attract. A professor of chemistry at Wayne State University, a Dr William F. Koch once stated that the main cause of free radicals in the body is a lack of appropriate amounts of life and health sustaining oxygen.

Nature has its own innate method of purifying the air we breathe by using Ozone's negative charge to attract the positively charged, nasty, hydrocarbon based air particulates or free radicals.

So, if ozone is such an efficient and effective treatment for disease, why is it so unknown and obscure? Most have never even heard of Ozone Therapy. Nikola Tesla had successfully experimented with it back in the late 1800's and early 20th century.

Ozone therapy was practiced and in use back in the 1920's and 30's but was unfortunately put out of business by the large up and coming drug company cartels. They were more or less in the business of destroying and dismantling anything that interfered with their highly profitable, patented, petrochemical based drug therapies.

They even set up a bogus medical doctor as editor in chief of their newly formed medical journal to discredit the use of oxygen as a therapy in the eyes of the public. They succeeded and changed the face of medicine and its schools of education over to the sole practice of allopathic, orthodox medicine.

They very cleverly and conveniently erased Homeopathic and Naturopathic medicine and initiated our dependence on heavy drugs, major surgery and extended hospital layovers.

They did everything they could to promote the practice of allopathic medicine. It didn't matter how many people died or how many ended up suffering an unnecessary fate brought on by the numerous side effects of the heavy drug therapies and radical surgeries. Alternative practitioners were either ostracized, slandered, put in jail or had their medical licenses revoked.

This practice has remained in place for far too long. The long standing worship and God like status of our illustrious allopathic physicians is finally weakening. Too many patients have lost their will and their energy to fight from the multiple drug side effects. They have also, sadly, depleted the majority if not all of their finances before deciding on an alternative approach.

There are numerous articles degrading Ozone and its harmful effects especially in relation to the respiratory system. There are even machines and remote appliances that claim to remove this toxic and harmful ozone from your home.

It's very convincing and a big selling point when they use fear to associate Ozone with smog and pollution then claim it is responsible for the irritation in your lungs, eyes and throat. They use this scare tactic about Ozone and its dangers to keep you focused elsewhere instead of focusing on the numerous factory smokestacks that are really to blame for your discomfort.

Ozone used in its proper proportions is an amazing air purifier and one of the safest medical therapies in existence. It causes irritation when the respiratory system is so overloaded with toxic pollution that the Ozone begins its healing response. It will initiate a detoxifying effect within the body. That's what it does. This is the main reason why it needs to be regulated by a trained medical practitioner so as not to oxidize wastes within the body and or the lungs to rapidly.

Ozone air purifiers are completely safe when properly regulated at home. Don't let the pundits scare you off. It needs to be slowly and methodically increased as your lungs become accustomed to it. Start off gradually and see what kind of response or irritation you have. Start by keeping it set on the lowest setting and go from there.

Initially you should set it up on the lowest setting on a day where nobody will be at home. It has an unpleasant smell as it oxidizes the contaminants and bacteria in the room. Once the room air has been initially purified, the odor will dissipate. Just be sensible as with anything that detoxifies the body and its component parts.

Oxygen actually stores the sun's energy so that everything living can feed off of it. A great majority of stress relieving practices are focused around the breath. The enormous and healing power of the breath. This stored energy is what is referred to as Prana, Chi, Ki or our life force. Ozone translated from the Greek means 'The Breath Of God.'

One of the greatest plagues afflicting man today is waterborne diseases. These diseases are caused by anaerobic microorganisms. The same microorganisms that cause the majority of diseases in animals and humans. If you remember, anaerobic means absence of oxygen.

The same is true for the majority of crop diseases and failures. This is caused by a lack of oxygen in the soil. Plants and crops rely on oxygen loving bacteria attached to their roots. These bacteria predigest nutrients in the soil and make minerals and other trace elements into an available form for the crop or plant to utilize.

Many commercial growers add oxygenating solutions to the soil or to the water they use to nourish and condition their crop. By adding oxygen, they lessen the chance of diseases destroying their harvest.

Farm and other commercially raised animals have been cured of a variety of potential epidemics and outbreaks by simply oxygenating their water supply and or adding oxygen supplements to their feed.

A Dr. Migdalia discovered that there were 2 forms of cancer, environmental (from irritants) and genetic (budding under proper conditions). His research also revealed that T-cells in our bodies produced ozone, an active form of oxygen, so if we put ozone into the body of cancer patients we would be in line and duplicating Nature's laws and attacking the cancer cells naturally.

Another researcher, Lee Devries, put human cancer cells on microscope slides and filmed them. The cells would lose their red color and turn green and die, all within 11 minutes. This was all based on the theory that cancer cells were plant type cells growing in humans. The cancer cells would start to grow under the light of the microscope but quickly died because their metabolized waste product, oxygen, produced by the T-cells, was trapped under the microscope slide.

This research was based on the observation that if you feed any organism its own waste product it will die.

A Mr. Seifer, who spent some time with Devries and later started producing air ozone machines, in 1985, received a call from a Dr. Johnson asking about ozone therapy for cancer. He gladly informed Dr. Johnson, the personal physician to President Reagan, all about ozone.

Our former President, very quietly went to Germany to Dr. Hans Neiper's clinic where he had his cancer cured by ozone therapy. At the same time doctors using ozone therapy here in the U.S. were being persecuted by the food and drug administration. Big surprise.

The German ozone physician, Dr. Hans Neiper stated, "I can't divulge all the names of the heads of the U.S. Government, the heads of your cancer institutes and the names of their friends who have come for ozone treatments at my clinic."

Oxygen levels are decreasing worldwide. There are some countries and even some states here in America where the levels of oxygen are severely limited. It all depends on the amount of industry and the types of factories spewing lung choking, toxic debris and hydrocarbons from their environmentally regulated smokestacks.

Anyway, there was a gentleman that measured the oxygen content in the area near Gary, Indiana where they have a plethora of steel mills, blast furnaces and a major pollution problem. This place really stinks. The oxygen content of the air measured 9-11%. Wow! We have shortness of breath when the oxygen content drops into the teens and below 7%, we cease to exist. Sure doesn't seem like they're very well regulated.

We have allowed the pollution in our cities to accumulate and with the environment so badly deforested and destroyed, our oxygen supply commonly drops below 21% depending on where you live. Thing is, we were designed to live on this planet with an atmospheric sea full of high level oxygen. Somewhere between 38-50%. Oops.

Our ancient ancestors lived in a very highly oxygenated environment and now we live with less than half or maybe even a third, depending on where you live, of what our bodies were designed to thrive on. This is ultimately where all of our health problems originate.

There is much less untainted, (not bound in pollution) energetic (high atomic charge) oxygen available to us and this lack is destroying our quality of life. The rest of our air is nitrogen plus trace elements of noble gases.

Oxygen is what gives us life and its what Nature uses to clean us out. It's a sad fact when there is not enough oxygen for our bodies to perform properly and efficiently. Our bodies are now filled full of dirty, filthy, contaminated and congested fluids.

So much of our oxygen is bound with pollution that our bodies are constantly crying out for good, clean, crisp, clear oxygen and water. It uses all the pain and discomfort and other warning signals along with chronic degenerative diseases and other afflictions to awaken us to the fact that something vital is missing.

The oxygen we breathe comes from 2 places, the plankton in the ocean and the growth of flora in our towns, mountains and forests. The light from the sun strikes the plankton and when energized with this light they produce oxygen. The sun's light stimulates the ground plants as well and they create oxygen as a waste product of photosynthesis.

It's something we really need to be concerned about. It is not some fixed amount of oxygen that just happens to be here. It is manufactured through our ecosystem and our environment daily, continuously and constantly. We are destroying its sources on a regular basis. Those environmentalists don't seem so wacko now, do they?.

There's a quote that speaks of the blue planet, in its waters, first life was born and plankton started producing oxygen from carbon dioxide. The oxygen was very important, it gave birth to the green plants, which slowly became the roots of our planet and produced even more life sustaining oxygen.

Then, together with the Earths magnetic shield, the oxygen protected its surface from the threatening solar winds. Humans draw energy from oxygen and glucose produced by the green plants, converting it into bio-electrical energy (ATP), CO2 and H2O. CO2 and water are then used by the plants to produce new glucose and new oxygen.

This is the circle of life and it must not be interfered with or broken. Without glucose and oxygen, our cells cannot function properly or produce enough ATP, and low cell energy results in cell damage or death. Nearly 98% of all diseases are caused or complicated by hypoxia, lowered concentrations of oxygen in the body.

In the last 100 years we have polluted our environment, polluted our air, poisoned our waters, cut and burned down trees and plants, and despite all the warnings, we have been expending enormous amounts of oxygen to provide energy for a more comfortable life.

How far will we go to maintain that comfort? How comfortable will you be when you kick up your feet in the recliner, switch on your favorite TV show, open a can of your favorite soda pop or beer but have problems catching your breath?.

There are several different ways of introducing extra oxygen into the body. For extremely serious and late stage cancers the RHP method is recommended. RHP (recirculatory hemoperfusion) therapy has been likened to a form of ozone dialysis.

It is administered with some very sophisticated and specialized medical equipment and needs to be performed by a trained medical professional. The patient's blood is mixed with ozone in a closed loop device which is outside of the body. The blood coming out of the patient is typically a dark to blackish red color. It is then gently ozonated and re-infused back into the body. The freshly ozonated (oxygenated) blood is now a bright cherry red.

The patient's blood leaves the body only momentarily, enters the chamber where it is completely cleaned, sterilized, purified and oxygenated before being recirculated back into the body. The beauty of this style of therapy is that the dead toxins and microbes are filtered out before being recirculated back into the patient.

This is a huge benefit as the rate of application may be increased exponentially. Other oxygen therapies are also very successful but they must be administered at a slower pace because of the dead and dying toxic debris. The other forms of oxygen therapy have to take into consideration the cleansing/detox reactions initiated by the ozone and oxidation of pathogens.

This RHP (recirculated hemoperfusion) style therapy saves the liver, kidneys and lymph systems from having to deal with dead microbes and inactivated toxins. This helps to maintain the patients comfort levels thus creating a greater willingness to stay connected to the therapy.

Because the cleansing reactions are extremely minimized by this ozone/filtration process, the speed of recovery and or healing is greatly advanced. RHP is the leading, state of the art, cutting edge treatment in oxygen/ozone therapies.

Unfortunately it is not a home based unit. The process needs to be monitored by professionals. It is highly effective for a whole host of afflictions including late stage cancers.

Mr. Oxygen, Ed McCabe, tells the story of an AIDS patient that was brought in to one of the clinics on a stretcher, nearly dead and unconscious. They figured he had nothing to lose so they decided to hook him up and see what would happen. Apparently after a few hours hooked up to the RHP, he eventually woke up and after a while ended up walking out of the clinic.

There are other ozone treatments available. The Germans have been using autohemotherapy for over 50 years. Autohemotherapy deals with the removal of small amounts of blood, usually 250-600ml, then ozonating that blood for several minutes and re-infusing it back into the patient by way of an IV drip. Unfortunately this system does not filter out the toxins but instead acts as a type of auto-vaccine for everything in the blood.

Another common method is direct IV ozone treatments. This involves direct injection of a specific quantity and concentration of medical grade ozone into the body. This method of treatment is considered the 2nd most effective after the RHP (recirculatory hemoperfusion) therapy. This has also been in use for well over 50 years.

The direct IV is superior to the autohemotherapy as the direct IV delivers a higher concentration of ozone into the body. It is also more affordable than the RHP or the autohemotherapy. Mostly because it requires less equipment.

The benefits and advantages of direct IV are: a very precise dose is administered, the cost is much less than other applications and it requires fewer applications, plus it has produced better results than autohemotherapy especially dealing with lung cancer, AIDS and allergies. It eliminates unwanted antibodies and microbial components that contribute to cancer, degenerative diseases, immune disorders, vascular diseases, allergies and other environmental illnesses.

The direct IV injection is more consistent than autohemotherapy and it immediately starts to react with any type of oxidizable substrates, including lipid cell membranes, viruses, bacterial infestations and fungi.

Our bodies are extremely smart and will suppress, cover up and inactivate any illness we have ever had with a layer of hardened, protective mucous. In other words, the body effectively walls off and suppresses the symptoms of the disease to keep it away from the rest of the body. We think we are cured when in reality, the body is still harboring the disease, it has just constructed a wall of mucous to protect it and us.

The ozone/oxygen will surely and methodically burn up this protective mucosal layer. This can and will typically bring about the original symptoms associated with that disease. This is the detox/cleansing response. It is uncomfortable but mandatory for your recovery.

Monitor your condition and adjust your dosages accordingly. If you are extremely tired and are experiencing cold or flu like symptoms, this is an indication that you are backed up with too many toxins and your body is unable to keep up. This is when you would typically back off the ozone injections and switch to an oral oxygen supplement to help keep the toxins in solution and at least moving.

This is when colonics or enemas (coffee) are very helpful, also drinking plenty of water along with light exercise (walking is good if you feel like hell) to keep your lymphatic fluids moving. The reaction you experience is typically associated with whatever your weakest link is or the symptoms of any long term affliction you may have been dealing with.

Other applications include intramuscular injections, varicose vein injections, direct injection into tumors and a very specialized practice called portal vein injection. There are also ear insufflations, rectal, vaginal and penile insufflations. A catheter is typically used for these type applications.

The Russians have developed a system of adding ozone to intravenous, drop by drop saline solutions. It is called "Parenteral Ozone" and it has also been proven to be very effective. The majority of the ozone therapies and their effectiveness is most often related to how much ozone can be safely and comfortably delivered intact, into the body.

Ozone stimulates the production of white blood cells and interferon levels are significantly increased. Interferons are globular proteins and carefully orchestrate every function of the immune system. Ozone has been proven to elevate interferon levels.

Ozone also stimulates the production of TNF (Tumor Necrosis Factor). TNF is produced when a tumor is growing and when and if a tumor turns metastatic and cancers cells start breaking off, TNF inhibits these cells from setting up shop elsewhere in the body.

Ozone also stimulates the secretion of Interluekin-2 which is also a huge component of the immune system. It is secreted by T-helper cells. The interluekin-2 then binds to a receptor on the T-helper which causes it to produce more Interluekin-2. It's main function is to induce lymphocytes to differentiate and proliferate, yielding more T-helpers, T-suppressors, cytotoxic T's, T-delayed's and T-memory cells.

Ozone inhibits the growth of new tissue. Rapidly dividing cancer cells shift their attention away from producing the enzymes they need to protect themselves from the ozone so, in essence the ozone inhibits this new growth.

It also oxidizes arterial plaque, clearing blockages of large and small vessels and enabling a larger volume of oxygen to reach affected organs. It also increases the flexibility and elasticity of red blood cells. This increase allows oxygen saturation to remain elevated for several days and even weeks after ozone treatment.

There are also ozonated pills, powders, lotions, drops, water and ozonated oil. The applications combining oxygen are growing more commonplace everyday.

Homozon is a powdered form of pharmaceutical magnesium and is used as a colon cleanser. Homozon is high grade magnesium with ozone bonded to it. There are many copycat products on the market but the majority do not compare to Homozon and the rich quality of their pharmaceutical grade magnesium.

The majority of the off brands trying to copy the quality of Homozon, use basic magnesium bonded to oxygen not ozone. Remember that extra molecule of oxygen that classifies it as ozone?

Apparently bonding a gas to a solid is some sort of trade secret. The creator of Homozon, a Dr. Blass reportedly lived in the same hotel as Nikola Tesla in NYC. Many think it was Tesla who helped Dr. Blass put together this binding formulation. There is reported to be a vast difference in quality and overall effectiveness of this particular product.

The use of Homozon can cause frequent and loose stools. This, as some will claim, is diarrhea because of the magnesium. This is not the case. The loose stools are the result of oxidizing solid waste from a clogged up, mucous filled, toxic colon. The loose stools will cease as soon as the digestive tract is free of this accumulated waste matter.

This is a very effective way of thoroughly cleansing the colon. In fact many of the new colon cleansing products on the market now claim to be oxygenating colon cleansers. Homozon is the original and reportedly the best on the market.

Homozon is another way of introducing oxygen into the body and clearing out your colon from years of accumulated build-up. Just beware, it works fast and you will more than likely pass some extremely foul smelling, alien debris.

Another method of delivering oxygen to your body is with ozonated oils. Olive oil is typically used because of its excellent ability to retain the ozone gas. It is usually used topically as it is easily absorbed through the pores of the skin which then enters the circulatory system and into the bloodstream.

Practitioners report that ozonated olive oil has been used successfully to treat: athletes foot, acne, bacterial infections, bed sores, blackheads, bruises, candidiasis, carbuncles, chapped lips, cuts and wounds, dandruff, dermatitis, eczema, diaper rash, earache, fungal infections, impetigo, insect bites, fistulae, gingivitis, herpes simplex, hemorrhoids, leg ulcers, shingles, spots, stomach conditions, sunburn, whiteheads, wrinkles and yeast infections, to name a few! Ha! Ok, a little more than a few.

Ozonated oil also aids in wound healing, improves blood flow and circulation and helps to alleviate pain and reduce inflammation. It can be taken internally on a daily basis if desired. Ingesting about ½ a teaspoon to 1 tablespoon will help to cleanse the liver.

You will want to pay attention to your bowel movements. Ingesting too much internally can loosen stools so start with a half a teaspoon and see how your body tolerates that amount. You can always increase it from there. It can be taken 2-3 times a day and has very beneficial and refreshing benefits. It's another one of those monitoring moments, pay attention.

There are many more different types of treatments and applications available. Is it safe? The majority of these treatments are illegal in the U.S.. Germany has and is the leading provider of ozone therapies. The German Medical Society reported that 384,775 patients were given 5,579,238 applications of ozone. The side effect rate was reported and observed at only .000005 per application. That's a lot of zero's I know but they are on the other side of the decimal point.

Anybody care to compare that with the drug interactions and side effects from modern chemotherapy and other related drugs used in the treatment of cancer and other illnesses? I didn't think so. Ozone administered by educated and responsible practitioners is very safe and most importantly extremely effective.

It is said that there are only 2 diseases, the one that a person has and the one he or she can eventually get. Which one will you succumb to? When do you take a stand and start caring about what you are sacrificing for your comfort, your environment and your children's quality of life?.

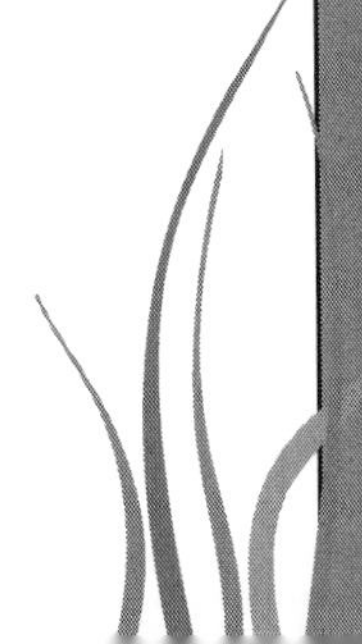

Chapter 8

The Gerson Therapy

There are a couple of doctors, actually quite a bit more than a couple, that commented on this therapy. They too were bewildered why the masses had not even heard of this protocol for cancer. They mentioned that it had cured some of the most virulent forms of cancer known to science. They were saddened that so many will perish never even aware that this therapy existed.

Statistics prove that we are living longer than ever before. This may be true but how are we living? Are we living longer in better health, free of symptom suppressing medications? Free of pain and chronic infirmities? I don't think we are.

Has the quality of life been enhanced for our aged and older generations or are far too many simply existing on multiple medications, coping with arthritis, dementia, Alzheimers, Parkinsons and other lifelong, enduring afflictions.

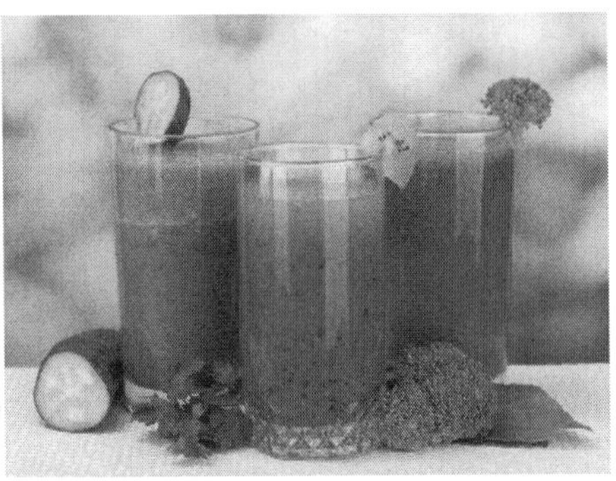

The Gerson therapy aims to bring us back to Nature, back to our roots. The roots of the Earth. This therapy does not address an isolated organ or symptom as if one part of the body was a separate entity from the whole.

The body is a machine, an amazing and miraculous engine of perfection. If you blow an O-ring somewhere in your car engine and oil and pressure start leaking out somewhere, it will eventually burn up a ring, a push rod, a piston, a valve, or whatever. Replace the O-ring first and then repair the burnt valve or piston or rod. We don't want it to happen again. You have to address the O-ring, the cause of the larger issue, the reason why the piston failed. You don't just surgically remove the piston. You have to repair the reason why the larger component failed. Simple whole, Holistic medicine.

We live in an allopathic, conventional world of relentless specialization. We have a specialist for everything. Allopathic, orthodox medicine does not consider the synergistic relationship of all parts working together as a whole.

Louis Pasteur, the 19th century French scientist maintained that diseases were caused by germs and that by destroying the germ the cure was achieved. Antoine Bechamp, his opponent, claimed it was the condition of the organism or the environment, not the germ that needed attention.

Pasteur later relented on his deathbed saying "the germ is nothing, the terrain is everything." A courageous and bold proclamation. He graciously relented his theory and gave credit to his long time rival.

This is the belief and goal of the Gerson Therapy, to restore the terrain of the organism and the isolated part that is afflicted will heal and cure itself. The beauty of this approach is simplistic and profound.

When you treat cancer and target the terrain of the whole body, the entire body will heal. You can't hold onto one disease and cure another when you address the whole organism. All afflictions will be affected.

Do not assume that this therapy is outdated. There have been some very carefully chosen improvements and accepted additions to the treatment since its inception close to 60 years ago.

The basic premise being fairly unchanged since 1958. Human physiology has not changed and the initiation and nature of chronic disease also, has not changed. Then again, I'm sure you could find someone to argue that point.

The protocols change accordingly. Pollution has gotten progressively worse, food grown in mineral deficient soils has also escalated. Chemical additives and preservatives are new and improved and have changed and grown evermore abundant in our western diet. This all adds up to a highly toxic, modern day dilemma of unhealthy lifestyle and food choices.

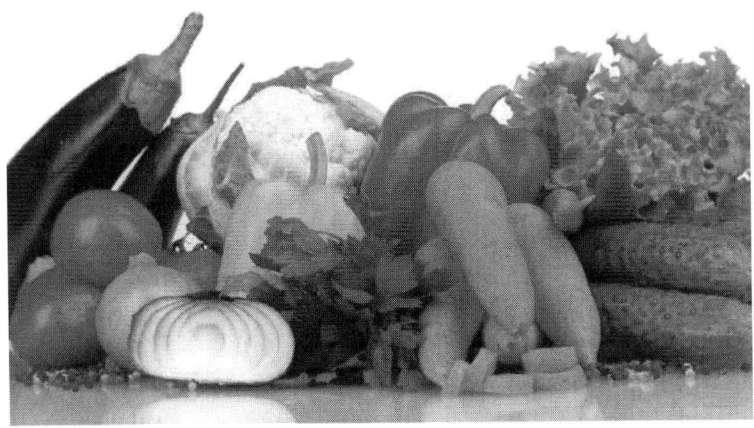

Many people have decided on the Gerson therapy simply because it was one of the few that actually made sense and offered the promise of a realistic, lasting cure. It focuses on the two major enemies of great health, toxicity and deficiency. Both being the by-products of an artificial society and a denatured way of life.

The quality of our air has deteriorated with way too many vehicles spewing exhaust, toxic aircraft residue, emissions raining down from what used to be crystal clear blue skies, chemicals from factories and toxic flatulence from our over cultivation and ever growing consumption of animal flesh. These are just a few that have contributed to our current quality of air.

We have our water contaminated with fluoride, chlorine, residuals from a wide variety of pharmaceuticals and industrial and agricultural pesticide runoff. These have all contributed to the quality and biodiversity of our rivers, streams, oceans and other waterways.

In this modern day evolution we have a constantly increasing supply of electromagnetic radiation and wavelengths coming from computers, cell phones, cell towers, satellite signals, microwaves and other electromagnetic sources bombarding us daily 24/7.

Since we have our own electromagnetic energies built into our anatomy, this can cause major interference and balance issue's within our own system. The incidence of cancer clusters in highly electromagnetic areas is worthy of reflection and pause. It has gone way beyond coincidence.

Then there is the deficiency issue with our mineral depleted soils. What we do receive from modern farming practices are NPK, nitrogen, phosphorus and potassium. Man discovered that these 3 were all that were needed to make plants grow. There is a huge difference between a plant simply growing and a plant growing vibrant and full of life giving minerals, vitamins and other life sustaining, essential nutrients.

Keeping it simple, right? The thing is we end up deficient in the other crucial minerals needed for our bodies to function properly, and literally for them to survive. Deficiency, it's like showing up for a baseball game with a pitcher, a catcher and a center fielder. Sure, we can still play baseball but nobody will show up to watch the game. You need the rest of the team.

The Gerson Therapy focuses on the interconnectedness of the whole, the immune system, the enzyme system, the hormonal system, our essential organs, and our absolute need for specific vitamins and minerals.

All of our functions rely on a carefully orchestrated internal environment working synergistically together. They never stop doing their job and their job is to keep you well and happy and thriving.

Dr. Max Gerson believed in giving the body what it generally received from our environment, mostly, crystal clean water and whole food before we started destroying our precious links to health and the health of the planet. Simple concept, simple to conceive, simple to receive, Occums razor in a hand basket. Unfortunately we have turned it into a never ending quest for a cure .

Dr. Gerson placed particular emphasis on enzymes. Pancreatic enzymes for example are typically able to destroy tumor tissues and cells because they are recognized as foreign. Their basic function is to digest proteins.

Since the standard American diet is so high in animal proteins, the majority of our pancreatic enzymes are used to break down these animal proteins and very little of them are available to destroy tumor tissue. This leaves the cancer cells free rein to roam, replicate and spread.

Adding significant amounts of digestive and pancreatic enzymes is a major part of the Gerson protocol along with toxin free, raw, fresh and organic foods to help alkalize and oxygenate the body and its cells to speed up the cleansing and detoxification process.

One of the main protocols of his therapy includes coffee enema's. They were and continue to be a mandatory part of the Gerson Therapy. I'll try and explain why they are so effective and beneficial.

...Gerson Therapy/Coffee Enemas...

To the uneducated, the use of enemas, especially coffee enemas, is an enigma. Some even laugh at the ridiculousness of using coffee as a healing agent.

The reason for it's use is the benefit to the liver. Since the fasting and or healing process initiates the destruction of diseased tissue, the liver can become overburdened and toxic. The liver is our main organ of detoxification. Its functionality is crucial to our recovery and lasting chances for a healthy life.

A cancer patient has, more often than not, already severely compromised their liver. If the liver is restricted or even somewhat comatose from toxic damage, chances of recovery are very slim.

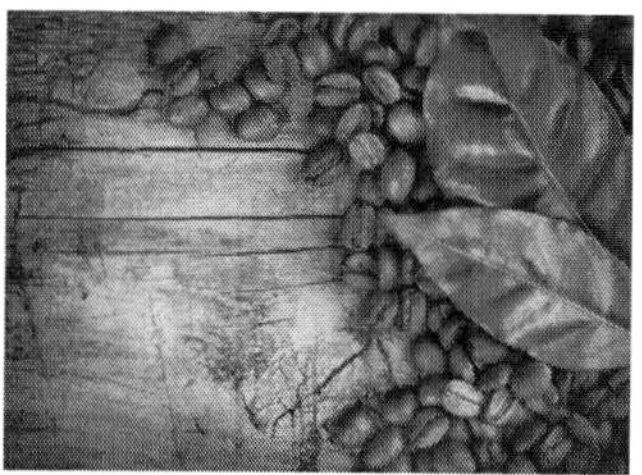

The "Father of Modern Medicine" Hippocrates, frequently prescribed enema's for many of his patients over 2,000 years ago. The revered Indian philosopher, Patanjali, also known as the first author of any written work on Yoga also recommended enemas for inner cleansing and elevated enlightenment.

One of the main protocols of the Gerson therapy is coffee enemas. Why enemas and why coffee? Will putting coffee up your butt in the morning stimulate your awakening the way consuming it via the normal route, your mouth?

That's a reasonable question. Most of the critics like to blast and besmirch the use of enemas period, let alone adding your favorite cup of Joe to the mix. Seems like a waste putting it up your back side when you could savor it with a nice crispy Italian scone. Once a patient decides on the full Gerson protocol the detoxification process begins as do the lattes up the butt.

Coffee enemas are one of the most controversial of all alternative procedures. It is very often used as a lead in to discredit or support the absolute insanity of alternative medicine and its claims to cure anything. It has become the butt of all jokes. Ha!

Believe it or not the earliest medical text in existence, the Egyptian Ebers Papyrus mentions its use. The Pharaoh's before that even had special doctors that would administer the royal enemas.

The Greeks often wrote about the cleanliness of the Egyptians. Enemas and emetics were a part of their internal cleansing systems. According to Herodotus these were administered on 3 consecutive days every month. The Egyptians believed that diseases were acquired by the superfluities of food.

Enemas were known by nearly all the ancient people of the world. Babylonia, India, Greece, China, Sumeria, South America and across Europe. It was also common practice among Native American Indians. In France it was common after dinner to administer an enema.

The use of enemas was practiced not only for its health benefits but was also practiced for its effect on your complexion. Heads up girls, maybe you can trash all your time consuming and expensive cosmetics and start on a daily enema regimen. The added benefit would be outstanding health and a beautiful complexion. I could use some of that myself.

When dealing with cancer your body and necessary organs need to be able to keep up with the removal and elimination of toxic debris. You run the risk of overburdening your system, especially your liver if it is unable to efficiently dispose of these poisons once they start breaking free.

Chances are your liver is already compromised and in a poor state of functionality or the cancer more than likely would not be there in the first place.

The use of coffee enemas in America started quite innocently towards the end of World War I. Nurses were short on morphine for the wounded soldiers so they administered water enemas for pain relief.

Being that there was always leftover coffee from the nurses constantly trying to keep the surgeons awake, the nurses surmised that the soldiers might get some type of pick me up or possibly additional relief from their pain if the coffee was added to their enema buckets. They decided that it couldn't hurt, we shall not waste.

The soldiers soon thereafter reported greater relief from their pain. This information was brought to the attention of 2 research professors in Germany where they discovered that the caffeine traveling via the hemorrhoidal vein and the portal system of the liver, opened up the bile ducts allowing the liver to relinquish accumulated toxic debris.

It was further researched and confirmed by an Oncologist from Graz, Austria, a Dr. Peter Lechner, in 1990. He confirmed the efficacy of coffee enemas after a 6 year controlled test on cancer patients. He also identified the 2 components in coffee that were responsible for its beneficial effects in detoxifying the liver, cafestol and kahweol.

Our entire blood supply passes through the liver every 3 minutes, the length of time one typically holds onto the infusion of coffee is 12 to 15 minutes. Toxic debris and poisons would then be deposited and released through the bile ducts due to the stimulating effects of the coffee.

Three scientists from the University of Minnesota confirmed that rectal administration of coffee activated an enzyme system in the liver (glutathione S-transferase) which initiates the removal of free radicals from the bloodstream. Results show the coffee increases the effectiveness of this enzyme by 600-700% thus greatly enhancing detoxification.

The coffee enema should not be confused with high colonics which typically fill the entire length of the large intestine under pressure. This pressure can distend the colon and cause damage. They are also very beneficial to the body but should be administered with care and understanding of the procedure.

They can also wash away vital nutrients, minerals, enzymes and beneficial bacteria necessary for proper digestion. The coffee enemas purpose is to open up the bile ducts allowing the liver to more effectively cleanse itself. It is critical for the liver to be able to keep up with the constant and continuous dying and dead cancer cells and other toxic influences.

The most popular type of enema equipment used by the majority of Gerson patients consists of a plastic bucket lined with measurements in ounces along with the rubber tubing and other attachments. It can be purchased as a package with all the component parts.

The main part of the enema process would obviously be the coffee which should be organic, medium or light roast, drip-grind coffee along with filtered and properly distilled water.

...What Type of Juicer...

The Gerson Therapy consists of nutrition and detoxification of your body. It is based around drinking raw fruit and vegetable juices and eating only organic, unrefined foodstuffs. They highly recommend a specific type of juicer although other types may be used depending on the severity of your affliction.

Gerson recommends the Norwalk Hydraulic Press Juicer. You can research the different types of juice machines. The Norwalk is quite expensive. Gerson recommends this press juicer because of the quality and richness of the juice it produces and the amount of nutrients preserved using this style application.

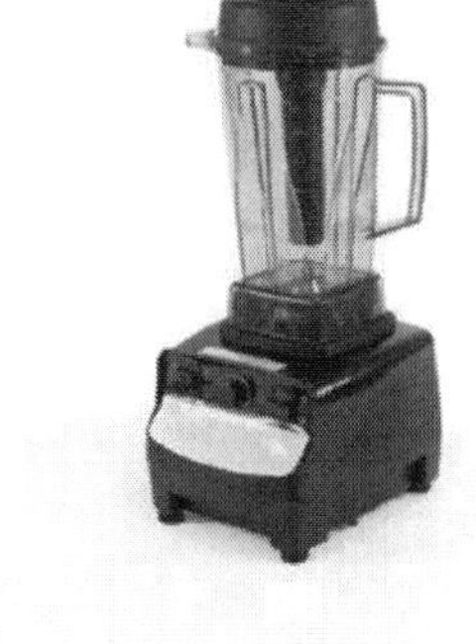

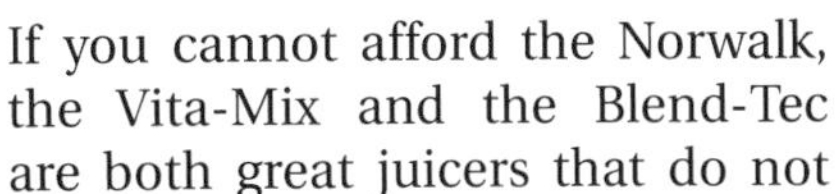

If you cannot afford the Norwalk, the Vita-Mix and the Blend-Tec are both great juicers that do not have a pulp separator. The biggest issue being the mechanism of action from a press or a centrifugal juicer. The centrifugal juicer, through its centrifugal action, introduces oxygen into the juice and partially oxidizes some of the nutrients.

...Scientific Research and Results...

So why and how does the Gerson Therapy work? It has been around for over 60 years and has a proven and reliable record of remission. Max Gerson died in 1959 under questionable circumstances. It's a long story but the fact that Dr. Gerson was having remarkable success curing what seemed to be incurable cancers quite possibly contributed to his questionable and untimely passing.

Since his passing, there has been some very credible research by very prominent scientists confirming his hypothesis. His protocol of supplementing potassium, restricting sodium, animal protein and fat proved to be legitimate and on target. Dr. Gerson's observations were curiously and unmistakeably correct.

An experiment carried out by a Dr. Robert A. Good from the University of Minnesota, also deemed "the father of modern immunology" expected to see a failure when he conducted an experiment using Guinea Pigs. One group he fed a protein free diet while the other group was fed the standard protein rich diet.

Dr. Good was quite surprised when his assumptions proved to be the opposite. The Guinea Pigs on the protein free diet had an extraordinary increase in thymus lymphocyte activity that remained quite active and aggressive for a considerable length of time. He had inadvertently stimulated the functionality of the immune system by restricting the intake of animal proteins. Weird, bizarre, and illogical, or so it was assumed. Hmmmm.

Dr. Gerson believed that the cancer patient would receive ample and adequate protein from the vegetable kingdom which is a large portion of the Gerson diet. After all, where do you think pigs, cows, and sheep receive their protein? They are all vegetarians, right? Last time I checked they were still not eating meat. That kind of puts a twist in your chain when you think about it.

There are a number of case studies where patients still received conventional, orthodox treatments but followed a watered down version of the Gerson therapy. What amount of the Gerson diet and protocol they followed is unsubstantiated since the protocol was administered at home. Regardless, at the end of 6 years the doctor who organized the experiment, Dr. Peter Lechner reported:

- Patients suffered fewer post-op complications and adverse side effects.
- Patients' mental and psychological state seemed to be more stable throughout.
- Patients' need for pain medication and psychotropic drugs was less than the control group.
- Cachexia, or severe wasting caused by malnutrition normally occurring in advanced stages of the disease, was avoided or greatly delayed in the majority of cases.
- A much slower progression of existing liver metastasis.

...The Do's, Don'ts, & Necessities...

There are thousands of people worldwide that have adopted the Gerson Therapy and put it into practice. Not only has it proven effective for treating cancer but any other malady that may be affecting your quality of life.

There are some do's and don'ts that need to be addressed since this is mostly a stay at home therapy. It's successes have been proven by many. The potential for your own success lies mostly in you. How diligent and how determined you are to follow the protocol precisely. It will take commitment and endurance. If you cheat, you only cheat yourself, there is no middle ground or benefit otherwise. The ball is definitely in your court, be patient and don't be afraid to take the open shot, let the games begin.

There is a highlight to the program that should help stimulate your perseverance. After the initial healing response has leveled out you will feel an amazing change in the quality of your health, your energy, and how you feel.

Your home needs to be turned into a place where you can heal. Toxic influences need to be addressed and removed. The microwave oven needs to find its way to the dumpster, if that is not possible unplug it and forget it exists. If you want more information on the dangers of microwave ovens and what it does to your food you can check out my blog and read the article, http://www.shockinghealthnewsletter.com/blog.

Stay away from aluminum cooking pots and pans and other aluminum utensils. Use only stainless steel, glass, Pyrex, or enameled cast iron pots. Use only stainless steel, wood, or silver spoons and other utensils.

Surprisingly, patients do not consume extra water on the Gerson diet. The protocol calls for 13 glasses of organic, freshly made juices, soups teas, and salads, which supply all the necessary liquids and or water needed. A home distiller is recommended for the water supply to make the necessary foods while on the diet, distilled water is also used for the enemas.

It is important to clean your distiller every 3 days as a significant amount of debris can build up depending on the quality of the water source. It's also important for the distiller to have a carbon filter which will further eliminate any volatile components. The myth that distilled water removes minerals from the body is just that, a myth. The majority of minerals found in water are inorganic and can prove to be harmful.

Be sure and stay away from any household items that contain chlorine. You can substitute chlorine based cleaners with malt vinegar diluted with water to clean kitchen surfaces or just plain soap and hot water. Just use common sense, stay away from any chemically laced products. Dishwasher soap, detergent and bleach need to be thoroughly removed from any of your washed clothing, a second rinse is advisable.

The premise is just to use common sense. When you are dealing with an affliction such as cancer, any and all chemical components within your control need to be avoided. Aerosol sprays, bathroom chemicals, chemically enhanced soaps, deodorants, perfumes, pesticides, paints, and anything else potentially toxic to the patient.

As caretaker and or spouse it is advisable and more or less in your best interest, to keep a tight and toxic free ship. Minimizing exposures that are within your control will contribute greatly to your healing.

There is a huge list of foods or what used to be foods that need to be avoided. These are mostly foods that man has cosmetically enhanced. Sugar substitutes like aspartame, Splenda, Equal, amino sweet, Sweet and Low etc., all need to be black listed. They are very cleverly disguised in over 5,000 different foodstuffs found in your local supermarket. If you want to find out more on the dangers of artificial sweeteners you can again read the article on my blog, http://www.shockinghealthnewsletter.com/blog.

All processed foods need to be avoided most importantly for their sodium content. Other banned foods to be avoided are any and all that have been commercially cultivated. They contain trace amounts of chemicals deemed supposedly harmless, like hormones, antibiotics, growth enhancers, pesticides, herbicides, fungicides, and all the other processed and fabricated toxins.

Some of the foods that are forbidden are a bit curious but need to be avoided nonetheless. This is all part of the Gerson therapy, ours is not to question why, the successes speak to the why. Here is the list of forbidden items:

- Alcohol
- Avocados
- Any and all processed foods
- All berries except currants
- Bicarbonate of soda in toothpaste, gargle and foods
- Bottled or canned beverages (Sodas)
- High sugar sweets like chocolate, cake and candy
- Coffee (Orally)
- Cheese
- Cocoa
- Commercial cosmetics, hair dyes etc.
- Cigarettes
- Cucumber
- Sulfured or glazed dried fruits
- I know it's odd, but no drinking water
- No Epsom salt baths
- No fats or oils except flaxseed oil
- No flour or flour products
- Avoid anything that may contain fluoride
- Only herbs permitted on the diet
- Ice Cream
- Milk
- Legumes (used later in the therapy)

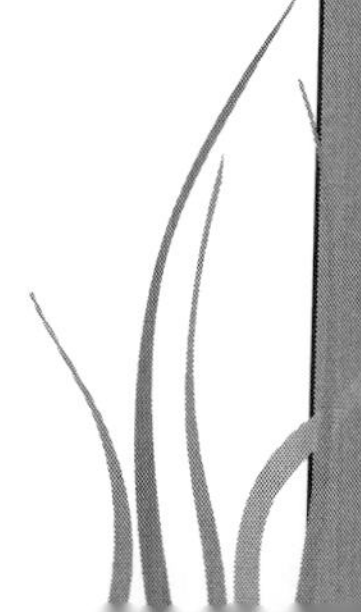

- Mushrooms
- Nuts
- Lemon or Orange rinds
- Pickles
- Pineapple
- Salt and any salt substitutes
- Soy or any soy products
- Most spices
- Sugar
- Tea
- No wheatgrass juice or sprouted seeds

There are other foods that are temporarily forbidden until a certain time in the treatment. Hopefully, if you have decided on this therapy you will have made contact with the Gerson Institute and will have an adviser and practitioner assigned to your treatment, progress and particular situation.

Someone at the Institute will be able to guide you through the protocol, keep records of your progress and let you know when other food groups may be allowed and introduced back into the diet. These foods include Cottage Cheese, Yogurt, Butter, Eggs, Meat, and Fish.

This may sound like hell on Earth, what's left to eat? Everything seems to be banned. We have grown so accustomed to eating foods laced with chemically addictive substances and heavy doses of salt that our taste buds are a bit confused. It will take a week or two before they re-generate their innate sense of flavor.

You will begin to start tasting the foods for what they are. We sometimes saturate our foods so heavily with sauces and spices the actual foodstuff itself is incidental. It is just a bulking agent used to fool the mind that we actually ate something. We just taste the spices, many of us have never experienced the true, rich flavors of cauliflower, broccoli or squash.

Preparation of the juices and meals on the diet are critical. It all must be organic, home grown if possible and fresh. The parts of the diet that are cooked must be cooked slowly using low heat so as not to destroy vital nutrients and enzymes.

Vegetables must retain their skins, so wash and or scrub them thoroughly. Remember that oxidation begins as soon as you cut into your fruit or vegetable so only start chopping and slicing when you are ready to begin cooking or juicing, then consume immediately.

The diet consists of a balance of cooked and raw foods. Dr. Gerson found that cooked foods were a necessary part of the diet. Given the amount of raw foods and juices on the diet, the cooked foods helped with digestion, eliminations and added soft bulk to the regimen.

There are only 4 different types of juices used in the therapy. Apple/Carrot juice, Carrot only juice, Green juice which consists of romaine, red leaf lettuce, endive, escarole, red cabbage, young inner beet tops, Swiss chard, a quarter of a small green pepper, and watercress. The 4th juice is orange juice.

Remember that your psychological state of mind is something that needs to be included in your therapy. This is a must with any therapy you choose. Find a mind-related, stress calming modality that works for you. Whether it be meditation, yoga, reiki, acupuncture, massage, or Qigong etc. Anything that will help keep you focused, relaxed and determined on your successful pursuit and outcome.

If you decide this is the therapy you are comfortable with, then you will need to contact The Gerson Institute or you may obtain information and material from their website. http://www.gerson.org/ to go to their website. Their address is P.O. Box 161358, San Diego, Ca. 92176 and their phone number is 619-685-5353

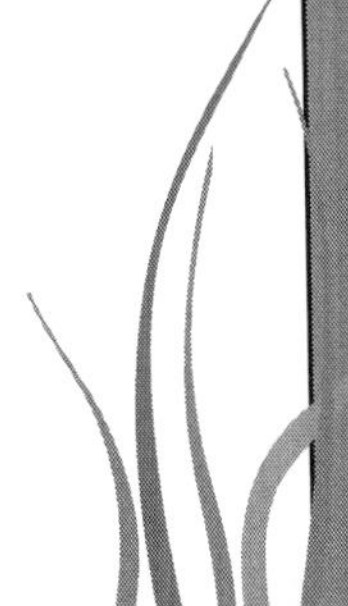

Chapter 9

Dr. Kelley & Enzyme Therapy

There was a cancer patient that detailed his personal account of this therapy to the state legislature where he lived. He apparently was sent home to die 7 years previously as conventional medicine had nothing left to offer. One of his doctors informed him that he had the fastest growing cancer known to man at the time and that their chemotherapy treatments would be of little to no help. In the end he remarked how he would have been just another cancer statistic had he not been directed to, and contacted Dr. Kelley.

A well known doctor commented that since the 2nd decade of the 20th century there has existed a compelling and very powerful cancer treatment. Enzyme Therapy---based on research by a Dr. Beard. He explained that this therapy was completely non-toxic, did no harm to the body and or it's organs, and is strikingly successful. This physician was confounded by the fact that this Enzyme Therapy was not perfected and made known around the world. He described it as one of the greatest mysteries of modern times, maybe the greatest of all time.

> "The person gets cancer because he's not properly metabolizing the protein in his diet."
>
> —Dr. Kelley DDS

This protocol was developed by a Dr. William Donald Kelley in the 1960's and 70's. The modality revolved around the administration of pancreatic enzymes in high doses. Initially proposed by a Dr. Beard in 1906. Dr. Beard believed that the pancreas was the key component in the bodies defense against cancer. This was based around the proteolytic enzymes typically secreted by the pancreas.

Oddly enough, years later, another Dr. Beard from Yale University expanded on the efforts and effects of pancreatic enzymes, (trypsin and chymotrypsin) and their effect on cancer cells.

It wasn't until the 1960's that a medical practitioner started treating cancer patients with pancreatic enzymes, (trypsin and chymotrypsin).

This is when Dr. Kelley began treatment on his own advanced, metastasized cancer and cured himself. Dr. Kelley was a practicing dentist when diagnosed with pancreatic, liver, and intestinal cancer.

The long term survival rate for advanced, metastasized cancer of the pancreas is around zero. Most newly diagnosed pancreatic cancer patients die within a year. Dr. Kelley was given only a few weeks to live and yet has remained cancer free for well over 40 years. He was obviously on to something worthy of exploration and investigation.

Dr. Kelley went on to cure thousands of cancer patients, and had the highest cure rate of any current, alternative medicine practitioner. He labeled his style of treatment "Metabolic Therapy." He classified each patient according to their metabolic type.

His therapy included: coffee enemas to detoxify the body and liver, (also an integral part of the Gerson Therapy), high doses of pancreatic enzymes, along with nutritional supplements, a nutritionally balanced acid/alkaline diet, physical, chiropractic or craniosacral therapies, and the all so powerful spiritual and or mental state of your mind.

He published a book that became very popular in underground, black market circles but was viciously harassed by the medical establishment. Eventually he was denied his freedom to expose and publicize his methods of treatment.

In fact, in the 1970's, a federal court ordered him never to write or speak about his methods or treatments again. This can't be real, right? They wouldn't let all our loved ones die unnecessarily if there was a cure or something that would lessen their suffering substantially, would they? Could they? Maybe the words ethics, integrity, or empathy hadn't made it into the dictionary yet.

They succeeded in keeping his therapies under wraps and from being exposed through the mainstream media. You wonder why you have never heard of the majority of these therapies? They are very good at what they do! It's called information control. It's a really big pill to swallow, but swallow we do!

Think of the implications of a simple pancreatic enzyme therapy and a change in your diet curing the incurable. No chemo, no surgery, and no radiation = no money. That's a lot of vacation homes and beach houses on the line for the pharmaceutical industry.

Dr. Kelley was more or less forced to pretty much disappear from the scene altogether. All a very closely orchestrated and precise conspiracy of confusion and illusion.

Dr. Gonzalez, a medical student from Cornell University at the time, was intrigued, and contacted Dr. Kelley in 1981. He examined his files and decided to study 22 of Dr. Kelley's most critical cancer patients. He chose the 22 because of their pancreatic cancer diagnosis and its extremely low cure and survival rate.

His results were nothing short of "this can't be right!" and total disbelief. How could this be? Surely the whole world would know of these discoveries, right? Surely this would be front page news across the globe. Every leading media organization would be leading with this Earth shattering, front page, medical breakthrough.

I'm sure you remember reading about it, don't you? Hmmmm, maybe I was too young at the time. Yeah, that must be it. Anyway.

Here are the results of his research: 10 of the 22 patients did not follow any of the protocols prescribed by Dr. Kelley and lived on average 67 days. 7 of the 22 patients followed some of the protocols prescribed by Dr. Kelley and lived on average 233 days. Interesting. 5 of the 22 patients who followed Dr. Kelley's prescribed protocols exactly experienced complete and total recovery. Hmmmmmmm.

A pretty simple approach to cancer therapy and the vital function the pancreas plays in the fight against foreign, cancer causing pathogens. It just seems too simple. But that's part of the problem, we have a hard time wrapping our minds around "too simple" sometimes.

Ever hear of Occums Razor? It is defined as: "the maxim that assumptions introduced to explain a thing must not be multiplied beyond necessity". I think it's like saying that sometimes simple wins the day and that by making something more complicated than it needs to be we miss the concept of what was staring us in the face the whole time. Sometimes we over contemplate and over complicate.

So many of the natural therapies run together, they are all pointing and leading us to the same conclusion. This is just another therapy where you give the body what it needs and used to get from our foods way back when, before we started introducing all these new, modern day, synthetic, foreign entities.

The coffee enema is a critical part of this therapy. I know I've mentioned the coffee enema several times throughout this book. That should be a huge clue as to how important and beneficial they truly are.

You can find out more information on Dr. Kelley and his Enzyme therapies. You can also purchase his book on figuring out your metabolic type. http://drkelley.info/ for his website. You can also check out his other website http://drkelleycancerprogram.com/.

He also has more detailed information on determining your metabolic type.

...Digestive Enzymes...

One definition of enzymes is that they are complex proteins that are capable of inducing chemical changes in other substances without being changed themselves.

All functions in the body require enzymes. The pancreatic enzymes are especially important in destroying tumor tissue because they recognize them as foreign. I know I'm repeating myself from an earlier statement in this book but when these pancreatic enzymes are so busy digesting difficult animal proteins they are way too exhausted to deal with destroying tumor tissue, therefore the tumor tissue propagates.

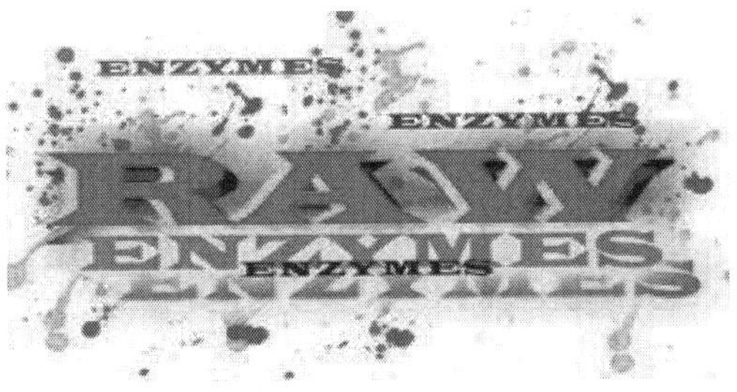

A Dr. Humbart "Smokey" Santillo made a statement that our modern day food enzyme deficiencies are our number 1 leading nutritional problem in America. He went on to say that this food enzyme deficiency was responsible for more infirmities and illnesses than any other nutritional inadequacies combined.

Another doctor stated that our lack of food enzymes and the result of that deficiency is the most profound and dangerous oversight in nutrition today.

When we ingest raw foods, the act of chewing actually releases the enzymes in that food and begins the process of digestion. You need to ingest and digest that last statement. "When we eat raw food" straight from the Earth and into our mouths, the enzyme process is put into play. Our nearly 100% cooked, broiled, fried, microwaved and boiled foods are slowly but ever so surely, killing us.

Why haven't we heard about the importance of enzymes? The majority of American's grew up on cooked foods. We still do. My mother would have been the first to demand we eat a certain portion of our meals raw. Enzymes are so important they should be a mandatory part of everyone's daily diet. We never gave the importance of raw foods a second thought. How much healthier might our generation be? What about the next? What about this generation? I think it's worse now.

Now that we are learning so much more about nutrition and what the body has to have to remain disease free, how will today's children fare? Not so good, in my opinion. I see firsthand what parents allow their children to eat. Can you identify the nutrients in the following daily diet?

Breakfast: Bowl of chocolate covered, peanut butter swirled, super, poofy puffs saturated with ultra pasteurized milk, oh, lets not forget to include a piece of processed cinnamon bread with vanilla frosting. Lunch: Processed cold cut sandwich on white bread with mayonnaise, a bag of special spicy hot chips, and an apple. Dinner: A whole, processed, frozen pepperoni pizza, and a frozen, processed, microwaved corn-dog along with a glass of ultra pasteurized chocolate milk. Hmmmm. Well? If you picked out the apple, you are correct. Whether or not they ate the apple or pitched it in the trash at school is unknown at this time.

What type of affliction or dis-ease could be growing inside of your child right now? What might be on its way once their enzyme supply is seriously reduced or diminished? Such a huge and simple fix. Such a profound contribution to your health and your health in the future. Seems we have programmed and endorsed the instant gratification persona. Planning ahead will always win in the end.

When I was a kid we used to love it when mom would make a huge salad with all the trimmings for a down home, cool, summer meal. That was the best. The reason why we never cried about having to eat a yucky salad or, went off on a major temper tantrum, was because we knew that whatever mom put on our plates for the evening meal was all there was going to be. If you wanted to eat, you ate what was put in front of you or you went to bed with a growling gut. No fights, no crying, no anger, no resentment. Eat or don't eat, that was our choice. The choice to eat was really popular at our house. Remember those days? I know, I'm old.

We never even considered that a constant and consistent withdrawal of enzymes from our body would be harmful somewhere down the road. We were surviving on a diet completely devoid of necessary enzymes. Almost everything was cooked. My parents certainly never knew how important these enzymes were.

If you think about kids nowadays, how many do you know that have ever eaten anything raw? I know, I can't think of any either. I guess an apple is the best we can hope for. The vast majority of kids in our modern society dictate to their parents what they will eat. Sadly, it's not the parents decision anymore. We gave them our power. We act as though these little monsters are better qualified to decide what their growing, maturing little monkey bodies need to survive.

I think we have just given in to giving them whatever they want to avoid listening to them wine and complain. Parents don't parent their children anymore. The kids somehow run the show. How did that happen, this sadly, ungrateful, twisted sense of entitlement? We need to take back our power and feed them what they need. What we decide and know they need.

Now that you know what a lack of these vital components can do to your body and to your kid's future body, what will you change? I know, your scared, your kids won't love you anymore if they don't get their greasy fast food burger combos, chicken nuggets, candy and ice cream So sad, so weak, so destructive down the road. I guess I can't blame a lot of parents, it's kind of just the way we allow it to be nowadays. We're to tired to fight them.

I am a new step-parent so I don't have much say so with anything yet, but I have 1 more sad but funny story. We went out to a buffet style restaurant the other day. You know the ones where you slide your tray along and pick and choose what you want to eat? This place was really well known for their soups along with a multitude of fancy salads. Of course they also had a vast array of baked, fried and sugar laced dessert foods.

My son finally settles down to the table with his dinner selections. He chose, chocolate frozen yogurt (only because they didn't have ice cream), 3 slices of greasy cheese pizza, blue jello, 3 chocolate chip cookies, chocolate milk, pudding, thank God an apple and 3 mini wedges of an orange. Yum! If you picked out the apple again and the orange wedges as the nutritional components, you got it right again.

Oops, sorry, how did I go from digestive enzymes to kids. Oh, now I remember. It was that talking about kids and how important it is to get them to eat some raw food. Remember there are no enzymes in cooked food. They need something that will help them stock up so they can make substantial enzyme deposits for their future digestions.

I almost blacked out at a restaurant the other day. Nothing fancy, so junk food was definitely available. I look over at this table and there are these 2 little girls. I would guess 1 was about 6 and the other maybe 8. They were both chowing down on a big, fresh, raw, mixed salad. No burger, no fries, no taquitos, no soda pop, no corn dog, just a big meal sized salad. I had to pinch myself. I figured I was hallucinating. They even had big smiles of satisfaction on their faces. It was almost as if they were enjoying it. What's up with that?.

A Dr. Edward Howell was a pioneer in enzyme research. In his earlier experiments he proved that a diet of cooked foods caused rapid and premature death in mice, and that the speed of the premature death was directly related to the temperature used during preparation of their cooked food.

A Dr. Paul Kautchakoff confirmed in his book that the effects of cooked food on our system included an increase in our white blood cells or leukocytes. This increase in leukocytes is necessary to transport enzymes to the digestive tract. Dr. Kautchakoff demonstrated that after a raw food meal there was no noticeable increase in leukocytes. By the way, that's a good thing.

The enzymes in raw food aid immeasurably in the digestive process. Their availability and action removes the stress of having to borrow from our enzyme reserves, especially from our white blood cells which are needed elsewhere in the body to support our weakened immune system.

Dr. Howell's studies concluded that the body has a finite enzyme potential or supply that gradually decreases as we get older. A Dr. Meyer and his associates found that the enzymes in the saliva of young adults was 30 times stronger than those in adults 70+.

Dr. Howell's research also concluded that the rate of enzyme depletion in the body was directly related to longevity. In other words, the more enzyme depleted foods you consumed, the greater the amount of enzymes your body would have had to acquire from your enzyme reserves, that is if you had any reserves left to borrow from. Pretty simple concept, pretty important component in your daily diet and hopes for a long life.

Could the lack of the appropriate enzymes necessary to digest certain foods be responsible for the indigestion you experience? Could this be part of the reason why certain foods don't agree with you? Maybe all you need is a good digestive enzyme supplement.

Enzymes initiate chemical reactions on our food. Digestive enzymes are produced mainly by the pancreas, stomach and salivary glands. The process begins in the mouth.

Enzymes in the saliva begin the process of breaking down starches and sugar molecules. Once it hits the stomach, hydrochloric acid begins the process of breaking down proteins while the enzymes in the raw food you just ate also assist in this process.

When we don't chew our food thoroughly, the enzymes in the saliva are unable to act before the food makes its way down into the stomach. From the stomach the food enters into the small intestine where enzymes secreted by the pancreas finish the digestive work until the nutrients are small enough to enter into the bloodstream.

Our enzymes are heat sensitive and are destroyed by our over consumption of cooked foods. As I have said before, this lack of vital, life sustaining enzymes have now been destroyed by our over the top, multiple and recreational cooking processes.

This puts a huge burden on the pancreas which, typically, in a well balanced raw/lightly cooked diet, finishes up the remnants of what was begun by the saliva and in the stomach. This increased burden on the pancreas can allow partially digested food particles to enter into the bloodstream.

This initiates an immune response attacking these foreign food particles because the body does not recognize them as nutrients, they're too big.

This response usually comes in the form of an allergic reaction or some type of inflammation. Your immune system then starts producing antibodies to fight the food particles instead of mounting an attack and fighting off real toxins. This also hinders healing responses elsewhere in the body.

Our enzyme supply and capacity changes over time as we grow into our golden years. It is also influenced by the foods we eat. The golden years are even more likely to cause reactions with certain foods as our enzyme supply is typically, by this stage in life, well overdrawn.

The moral of the story is "you absolutely, unequivocally, without a sliver of a doubt" have to have the proper enzymes for your body to endure. Endure gracefully into old age. Age gracefully with endurance. It's such an incredibly huge part of nutrition. Now you know how important these enzymes really are and all the infirmities and indigestion problems a lack of these digestive enzymes can create. They are the basic nuts and bolts of our existence.

You shouldn't just try and live with the fact that certain foods don't agree with you. If you have to take one of the OTC or, better yet, prescription, symptom suppressing medications an hour before you eat anything, try and figure out why it doesn't agree with you? Don't cover it up. Don't hide from it. You have a really good guess as to what might be the problem now, right?

Has your doctor ever, ever asked you if you were getting enough enzymes in your diet? Has he or she ever asked you if you were eating a good amount of raw foods everyday. Has your doctor ever recommended you take a full spectrum, digestive enzyme supplement? No? I'm not surprised. If you fix yourself you won't need the doctor and that's not good for business.

It really has a very substantial impact on how well you age if you are lucky enough to age at all. Ever notice how incredibly well some people age and others look absolutely horrific? They are the same age and neither one of them was ever a heavy smoker or a heavy drinker. What happened? Why does one of them look so good. You know the ones where we're dying to know their secret. Could it be? Hmmmm.

Could it be as simple as having enough and the right type of enzymes? Scientists, researchers and many doctors know that we are born with an enzyme potential, a certain amount in an enzyme bank account. If we go through life rarely making any deposits but, quite regularly, making withdrawals, what's going to be the state of that account when we are 50? 60? 70? Eventually that account is going to bounce. I know you've heard of overdraft protection, go eat a salad, make a deposit.

Maybe the people that look so good were making enzyme deposits all along so they never put that extra stress on their body? It puts a tremendous burden on the body and its organs when it has to go through life without enough of something so crucial.

Something to definitely consider. Too many people today survive solely on cooked foods. Eating something raw just doesn't work for them, well, sad to say it doesn't work for your body either. In the end, you ultimately should have payed more attention. Because someday, someway, something unwelcome, something unexpected will come to collect.

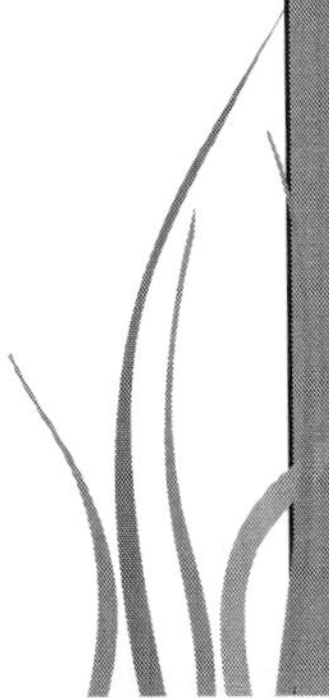

Chapter 10

The Hoxsey Therapy

The Hoxsey therapy is another natural, herbal approach to treating cancer. These herbal remedies and modalities have been around and practiced for thousands of years by indigenous peoples and tribes around the world.

It is by far the oldest practiced and the least understood. Probably least understood because it is not studied or funded commercially. Herbs cannot be patented so no-one is interested in putting up the funding or monies to study them. Simply because it wouldn't benefit anyone monetarily. Since they can't put their name on it as a patented product, interest is stifled.

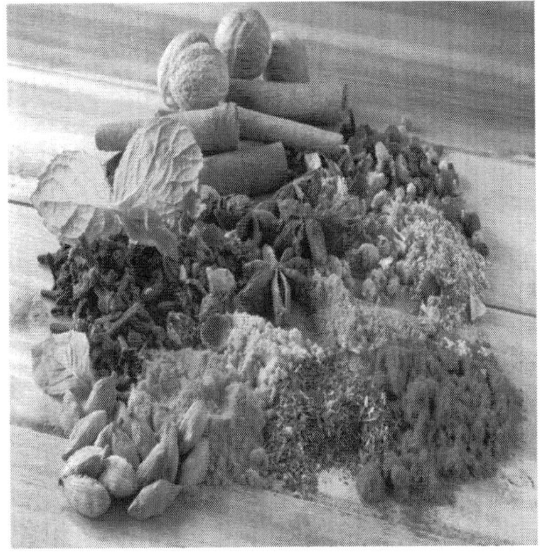

This is another modality that focuses on the bodies innate and inherent ability to heal itself with the proper ammunition and or nutrition. I think it's partly about believing that God designed our bodies and created the resources and food supplies to keep us in perfect health. I mean why wouldn't He. Our food supply is a very important if not the most important aspect of the bodies ultimate tool box.

Since so many things have been added or removed from our toolbox, disease has gained a foothold. What herbs do, being a whole, unmodified foodstuff, is replenish the tool box with the missing parts or components vital for our survival.

I don't believe any virus, bacteria, or cancer cell could survive if our bodies had a full and complete toolbox of ammunition, namely vitamins, minerals and essential fats.

The beauty of herbs is that for all their cancer, microbe destroying properties, they will not harm, kill or disfigure healthy cells, even though many act as strongly as commercially created pharmaceuticals.

The Hoxsey Therapy is a prime example of Natural Herbal Medicine. Many people have never heard of this therapy, although, it is the oldest, non toxic treatment for cancer in the U.S. or should I say used to be in the U.S. They have since been forced out of the U.S. and into Mexico. The treatment consists of a topical salve, a topical powder and an internally ingested herbal tonic.

It's recorded use dates back to the early to mid 1900's. The Hoxsey therapy treated thousands of patients successfully and had its largest facility in Dallas, Texas.

It was a remedy passed down to Harry Hoxsey from his great grandfather, John Hoxsey, who was a horse breeder back in the mid-1800's.

It's an interesting story how this remedy came to be. Turns out John Hoxsey had a horse that developed a cancerous lesion on its leg back in 1840. This horse happened to be one of John's favorites so, when he was forced to be put out to pasture, John made sure to keep an eye on him along with his other daily activities.

After several times of watching his horse, he noticed that the horse spent an unusual amount of time in a particular area of the pasture, a particular patch of shrubs and wild flowering weeds and plants.

The vet had informed John that this cancerous lesion was incurable and that the best thing he could do was to keep his horse quiet and to monitor it's progression. After some time out in the pasture, John happened to notice that the cancerous lesion had disappeared. It was gone. Somehow, someway the horse had made a complete recovery from this incurable cancerous lesion.

He was intrigued as to how this could have happened. He remembered the horse spending a good deal of his time in a particular area of the pasture. The story goes that he ended up collecting the flowering plants and herbs from this particular area. Then, out of curiosity, he decided to show the plants and herbs to some of the local Native Americans. He asked how they could be made into some type of herbal preparations. He then decided he would make an herbal salve, powder and a tonic.

His herbal preparations were having such great success treating other horses in the area that word spread and breeders were coming to him from miles around.

In order to keep helping and treating other horse owners and breeders, the formula was passed down to John's son who was a veterinarian. He began treating not just horses, but other animals with cancer and other afflictions. The successes continued to grow.

He also started experimenting on people with cancer who had been dismissed by conventional medicine and left without any other hope. They came to him. This was a very closely guarded experiment and the formula proved to be very successful on people too.

Harry Hoxsey at the age of 8 began helping his father. They began treating more and more people who were left with no other avenues from their conventional doctors. Just before his father's death, Harry was given the secret formula and continued with his father's work, treating people with cancer. The therapy was administered in private as Harry was not medically licensed to dispense medical advice, medicines, or treatments.

Harry decided he wanted to obtain the medical license to administer the therapy legally, so he started saving to help put himself through medical school. It seems the word had spread and while Harry was working to get his medical degree he was constantly being asked to treat terminally ill cancer patients who had nowhere else to go.

Being a kind hearted man, he eventually gave in and started offering the remedy to those who were desperate for his help. It wasn't until later that Harry found out he would be denied admittance into medical school simply because he was offering a remedy for cancer without a license. This threatened the all too powerful cancer establishment.

Luckily for Harry, or should I say his patients, a physician mentioned he could administer his remedies under the discretion of a licensed medical doctor, only if Harry was working as a medical technician under him. This was an ideal situation and the remedy continued to be very successful. Its success brought with it a following of desperate cancer victims.

When Harry was just 23 years old he opened his clinic in Dallas, Texas. It was the largest private cancer treatment center in the world. This was fully functional up into the 1950's but, with Harry not being a full fledged medical doctor, he was constantly being arrested and put in jail for practicing medicine without a license.

He always administered his treatments under the supervision of a licensed medical doctor, even so, it is said that he was arrested more times than any other person in the history of medicine.

Apparently the head of the AMA (American Medical Association) was out to get him. Mainly because Harry refused to sell him the secret ingredients for his formula.

The head of the AMA, Morris Fishbein was also the editor of JAMA (Journal of the American Medical Assoc.). Fishbein wrote several articles discrediting Hoxsey's formula as pure quackery. They also did their best to discredit any physician who stood by and supported the efficacy of the treatment.

It soon became professional suicide to be associated with Harry Hoxsey and his herbal cancer treatment. His arrests and incarcerations fortunately did not last long.

The success of the therapy brought along with it a whole host of cancer survivors and supporters that would lobby outside the jailhouse. They would bring Harry homemade food and sing hymns outside the jailhouse where it would annoy the warden enough to hasten his release.

They also had a hard time serving him arrest or court ordered summons. Turns out there were deputy sheriffs and or family members who had been treated and cured with his therapy. Ironically, in his court cases, many of the jury members had been treated or had family members who had been successfully treated by Harry.

The assistant district attorney had Harry arrested over 100 times. He viciously went after Harry for practicing medicine without a license until his own brother contracted cancer. His brother suffered through all the conventional protocols and eventually, like many before him, left without any hope.

At this point, the assistant district attorney's brother secretly went to Harry to be treated. The ADA drastically changed his tune when he discovered that his brother, who had been given up by conventional medicine, had fully recovered through the Hoxsey protocol.

The greatest irony of them all is that he later became Harry's attorney and began defending him in court. Funny how life throws you a curve ball every now and then. You either have to swing and risk striking out or get the heck out of your own way.

There was a nurse trained in conventional medicine that tried desperately to talk her own mother out of going to this quack, Harry Hoxsey. Her mother had been diagnosed with uterine cancer.

She had been treated with twenty units of x-ray radiation and thirty-six hours of radium. The poor woman was so badly burned from the radiation it took a whole year after that before she could pull a sheet over her body by herself in bed. She had wasted away to 86 pounds, was bleeding internally, and had to learn to walk all over again. Then her cancer came back.

This poor woman was told by her allopathic physicians that there was nothing more that could be done for her. The prognosis was terminal. It was then that she finally decided to try, against her daughters best advice, the Hoxsey therapy.

As hard as it is to believe, this poor woman completely recovered and died at the age of 99, 50 years later. She had outlived all the doctors and nurses that had treated her with conventional therapies.

The daughter, being a nurse, was finally convinced, especially after her father was diagnosed with cancer and would also completely recover through Harry's treatment. She then went to work for Harry at his clinic.

After many years of successfully treating cancer patients, even after an independent group of 10 doctors from across the U.S. concluded that the treatment was in fact successful and worthy of international attention, the powers that be, the powerful and burgeoning cancer/chemo industry sought to discredit and suppress their findings.

The compassion and gentleness of Harry Hoxsey needs to be noted. He obviously was not in this business for the profits. He treated all who came to him. It didn't matter if they spent their last dime on bus fare to reach the clinic, he accepted all who came to him.

Harry Hoxsey treated anyone in need of his services. Hoxsey claimed an 85% cure rate for external cancers and an 80% cure rate for internal cancers that had not already been treated with chemo or radiation.

Somewhere around 1960 the Hoxsey Cancer Treatment Centers were forced to close their doors. Former patients were intimidated by the powerful cancer machine and the propaganda campaign of his treatment being pure quackery, won the day.

The nurse who at first denied the efficacy of Harry's treatments who later started working for him, moved the operation to Mexico and continues the therapy to this day.

The hugely powerful cancer industry made sure that Hoxsey's simple, herbal, alternative treatment for cancer remain in obscurity.

The mainstream public was denied information and access to this remarkable treatment. The Hoxsey clinic is still operational as of this writing and is located in Tijuana, Mexico.

The ingredients in the tonic are fairly well known. Most sources claim it contains potassium iodide, licorice root, red clover, burdock root, stillingia root, beriberi root, poke root, casgara sagrada, prickly ash bark and buckthorn bark. The external tonic and salve contains bloodroot along with other natural herbs.

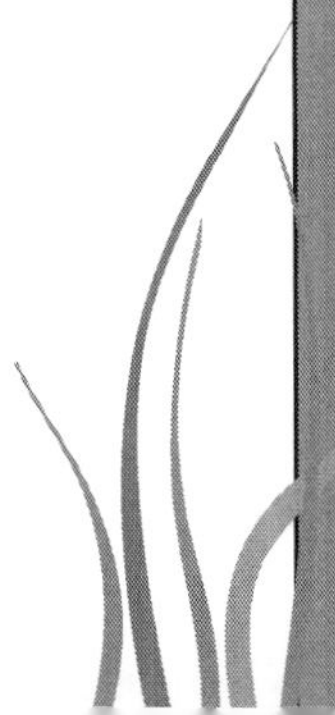

Chapter 11

The Rife Machine

This particular treatment some have said was the most effective treatment for cancer ever developed. Somewhere around 1930 an American scientific genius by the name of Royal Raymond Rife developed an audio frequency emitting device that targeted and destroyed cancer cells.

During his studies to become a medical doctor Rife became interested in the specialized field of bacteriology. He was soon after awarded a stipend from a businessman to pursue his studies in Bacteriology. A number of other wealthy businessman who also believed in Rife's abilities and vision also contributed. This allowed him access to a fully equipped laboratory for his experiments and research.

This is where he began his work in bacteriology and microbiology. There he went to work on his idea and vision that everything in existence vibrated at a certain frequency and that by electrically stimulating micro-organisms at a specific frequency, he could alter or destroy them. His initial experiments were very successful using audio frequency stimulation.

His ultimate goal was to include the study of viruses. He only had one small problem. Microscopes at that time were very limited in their magnification capabilities. The virus was too small to study under the current standard, scientific microscope. In 1920, Royal Rife developed a new design and style of microscope that was able to magnify over and beyond the current standard, thus enabling him to study his viruses .

This allowed him to see and categorize micro-organisms that had never before been seen. By the time he was finished, he had devised a microscope 8 times more powerful than anything in use by current day physicists.

Rife believed that cancer was a viral type organism. In 1932 he discovered two forms. One that caused carcinomas and one that caused sarcomas. He also discovered that this viral type organism was pleomorphic. Meaning it could take on different forms. In one form it was cancer causing, in the other form it was not.

Louis Pasteur and Pierre Bechamp were the leaders in this field in the 19th century. In fact Pasteur plagiarized many of Bechamps greatest ideas. It was on this particular subject that they were at opposite ends. Pasteur believed that these microbes were distinct and could not change throughout their life cycle.

French scientist Pierre Bechamp believed that the microbe could change forms. In fact, drastically, during its life cycle. He believed these microbes could change depending on the condition and health of the host organism or environment in which they lived.

It still remains a topic of debate for many scientists. Royal Rife was able through his discoveries to prove them to be pleomorphic. Eventually Rife was able to identify four distinct forms that this cancer causing organism could take during its life cycle.

He was actually able to initiate and complete the cycle from a virus to cancer, and from cancer back to a virus, all under microscopic examination. This was something other scientists were not able to do at the time but was later verified by other microbiologists who visited his lab, and were able to see his experiment firsthand.

Rife was a very well known and prominent microbiologist. He was awarded several grants. He was also written up in many magazines and newspapers and collaborated with many other well known doctors in their fields of study.

Rife's mission was not only to study and reveal these cancer causing, viral like organisms, but to find a way to destroy them. He experimented with a broad variety of audio and light frequencies.

He used only sine waves which are pure tones and frequencies, and they are also a single frequency.

Rife could literally see the viruses moving around under his microscope. He would then briefly zap the organism with the correct frequency and literally watch them die. The problem he now faced was breaking through and delivering the frequency through soft tissue and into living organisms, a challenging feat to say the least at the time.

Rife then, through experimentation, piggy backed this cancer killing audio frequency onto another frequency that could and would penetrate deep tissue. These two frequencies travel together but remain distinct and separate from one another. These he termed carrier frequencies.

In 1934 they set up a committee of leading medical doctors to oversee a human cancer trial. They treated terminally ill cancer patients who had no other hope for a cure. Within 70 days of treatment this committee announced 14 out of 16 terminally ill cancer patients cured. After another 60 days of treatment the other two of the original 16 were also cured.

With this successful treatment now documented, other doctors obtained the same apparatus to operate in their own clinical settings. They claimed an impressive and successful cure rate of 90%. Pretty impressive numbers. You would think that this discovery and the results would have hit every news media source worldwide.

There were virtually no side effects unless it was administered at too fast a rate, meaning, the dead cancer cells could not be eliminated fast enough and efficiently enough within the patients body. It was non-toxic and caused no healthy tissue damage whatsoever. Hmmmmm.

Naturally, the success of this device aroused unwanted attention, namely from the illustrious Morris Fishbein, the head of the AMA. Remember him from the Harry Hoxsey story. Well, not surprisingly, here's Johnny, I mean Morris, back on the scene.

Fishbein was trying to take control of the Rife technology for his own financial gain and offered Rife a small royalty for his invention and his apparatuses. Apparently Fishbein's offer was a bit questionable and when Rife refused, Fishbein set out to destroy Rife's newly formed Beam Ray Corporation.

The AMA filed lawsuits against the corporation and it soon went bankrupt as a direct result of these legal entanglements. Other businessmen became involved looking for profits and sadly, modified Rife's original design in the hopes of turning a quick profit.

The new machines did not produce the same impressive results as Rife's original design. In the meantime the AMA (Fishbein) continued to put pressure on doctors who were using Rife's invention. They cautioned them rather forcefully not to use this technology anymore in the treatment of cancer.

In fact they were threatened by the AMA to either stop using the frequency generators altogether or risk having their medical licenses permanently revoked.

Even today, the leading scientists in physics, microscopy and cancer research try to explain that suppressing a cure for cancer back in 1930 would have been impossible. Too many people would have known about it. Unfortunately, that same mentality persists today with not only the scientific community but the majority of the populace. How could something so astronomical and so monumental as a cure for cancer, be suppressed and kept quiet? But, kept quiet it was and it continues to lurk in the shadows.

When penicillin and other antibiotics came onto the scene they pretty much took away the interest and attention of the medical community. Fishbein and the AMA used their influence to promote the extraordinary notion of fighting disease with these new and exciting modern day wonder drugs.

Royal Rife agreed with Pierre Bechamp's original theory, that the cancer causing micro-organism is inside each and everyone of us, but it is the condition of the inner environment or host that determined and influenced whether or not it would devolve into a form that could cause cancer. In other words, "the environment is everything."

The concept of monomorphism still reigns in many modern day research facilities, although, other institutions have reportedly or should I say un-reportably verified the existence of pleomorphism. This ideal would support Rife's discoveries and give credence to his theories. Can't have that, especially when no one that matters or thinks that they matter, profits.

Bechamp believed that micro-organisms could change their shape as well as their size. His theories have since been confirmed, that contrasting types of bacteria were actually only a different representation of a bacterial collective. Many even say that the face of modern medicine would have changed dramatically had we followed in the footsteps and theories of Pierre Bechamp instead of the flawed ideologies of Louis Pasteur. Earlier acceptance of pleomorphism in the 20th century may have affected the outcome for the millions of lives lost to cancer.

Funny how the majority of people believe that modern medical breakthroughs are based on true and exacting science. Is it funny? I think not. There is way to much evidence to prove otherwise. But which holds the greater good for the bottom line, sad but true?

There is a great deal of medical science, sad to say, that is based on professional biases and the incredibly powerful profit margins of big business. You step on their wallets you cease to exist. It's part of the secret society. No, I'm not an extreme, conspiracy theorist. I'm just a realist with a conscience. Many government agencies are only a front so we can pretend we have a voice. There's no such thing as a true, dyed in the wool, democracy. It all comes down to "He who has the gold," always has been, always will be.

There are new Rife machines available on the market. How close they come to Rife's original design is questionable and unknown. The treatment is very simple and very basic. As with all the other therapies, administering the protocol at a reasonable pace and not to rapidly is highly recommended and just good common sense.

Dead tissue and dead cellular debris needs to be able to find its way out of our bodies. The channels of elimination need to be addressed and functioning well. Working any of the therapies at too fast a pace, more than your system is able to efficiently dispose of raises the risk of having these toxins recycled back into your bodily fluids, and causing uncomfortable and harmful side effects.

If you want more information about the Rife technology, you can check out a book by a very courageous author called "The Cancer Cure That Worked." by Barry Lynes. His information is very detailed and very accurate. There is also some really great information by a Dr. James E. Bare, D.C. He gives a summary of Royal Rife's resonant frequency therapy along with videos and information about building your own device. http://www.rt66.com/~rifetech/ to visit the website.

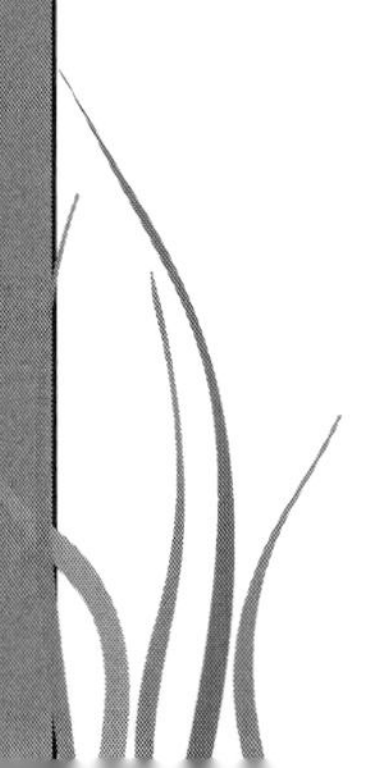

Chapter 12

The Photon Protocol

The Photon protocol is recommended for anyone who has very dangerous tumors, very advanced cancers and is extremely weak. This device can be purchased through the Ed Skilling Institute. A consultation with someone at the Ed Skilling Institute is required. They will recommended a nutritional protocol, specific to your type of cancer that will help deal with the type of microbe responsible for your weakened and ineffective immune response.

This protocol is based on re-balancing and re-building the immune system which, in the end, will be what keeps the cancer from returning. The Photon Genius Protocol is an electro-medicine protocol and is explained completely through the Ed Skilling Institute. This is probably the most powerful treatment available in electro-medicine.

The Photon Genius Protocol also utilizes the healing power of Harmonic energy transmissions using noble gases (Krypton, Xenon, Neon, Argon and Helium) transmitted with newly developed energetic, infrared wavelengths. This treatment targets the entire body and its parts.

It is very easy to use and has proven to be completely safe. It is a fairly large device measuring 6 feet tall, 5 feet wide and has 24 glass tubes and 60 infrared panels.

It effectively accelerates the power and effectiveness of the immune system. It helps to detoxify and clear congested areas of the circulatory system including the lymphatic system, blood vessels, arteries, capillaries and other pathways. These pathways are necessary for the delivery of nutrients, energy and communications throughout the brain, the body, cells and the nervous system.

The Photon Genius helps to dissolve mineral deposits, clots, blockages, lumps and other obstructions by re-polarizing cells. It effectively devitalizes harmful pathogens including; viruses, bacteria, parasites, fungus, yeast, mold and candida. It will reduce and or reverse disease processes in the body including, stopping any infections from progressing.

The Photon Genius device not only re-establishes the harmonic and vibrational frequencies of the cell but, produces powerful antioxidants, neurotransmitters and arterial wall relaxers. It is able to do all this through electromagnetic frequency generation.

The cells of the body communicate through electrical impulses from thought to intelligence, healing, pain, pleasure, self-awareness and consciousness.

All electrical fields create a corresponding electromagnetic field which can now be measured with our current, modern day instrumentation. How do you think an MRI (magnetic resonance imaging) generates its images? Science has also proven that normal cells have a higher magnetic resonance than abnormal cells.

The Photon Genius is able to provide re-vitalizing and nourishing electro-magnetic energy in a variety of different frequencies. These individually controlled frequencies allow The Photon Genius to affect the full spectrum of electro-magnetic frequencies within the body.

The Photon Genius also deals with Bio-Photonic energy (cellular light produced from our DNA), frequency harmonics, energy infrared transmissions, proprietary noble gas technologies, heat therapy, sauna therapy, anti-oxidative therapies, light therapies, sound therapies, nitric oxide therapies and more. It really is an amazing breakthrough in technology.

Since this is not a science book I will not get into the confusing and technical verbiage describing its applications. I just wanted to give you a brief but somewhat detailed description of this very powerful cancer treatment technology. Actually it is not only effective for cancer patients but for anyone suffering from any immune system dysfunction. The vast majority of any, and all illnesses and diseases are directly related to the quality and efficiency of our immune system.

The healing capabilities of this device and how it can transform your health is beyond believing. The Photon Genius is by far the most versatile, the most effective and the most powerful electromedicine device on the planet. Because of its multiple functions dealing with frequencies, photons, sounds, light, heat, infrared and noble gas technologies, it is rather expensive. As of this writing it costs around $25,000. Well worth the investment if you can afford it. If not and you would like to try this particular device, you can contact The Ed Skilling Institute http://www.edskilling.com/ for information on someone who may have the device for outside use, and for more information on the Photon Protocol.

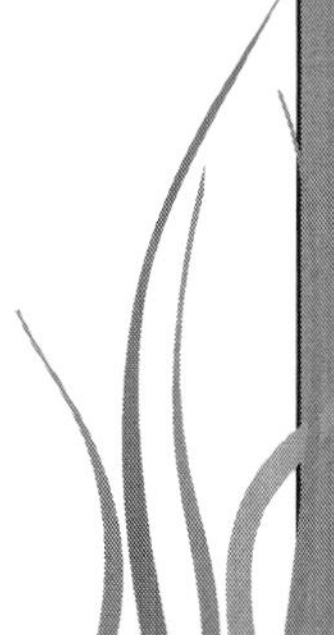

Chapter 13

Cellect Budwig Protocol

The Cellect-Budwig protocol was specially designed for advanced cancer patients. These are patients that need a therapy to become effective right away. They do not have the luxury of time.

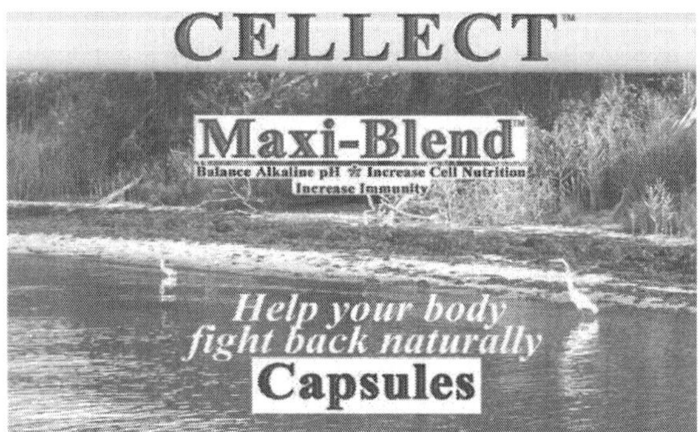

Not only are these very fast acting protocols but they cause little to no swelling or inflammation. These 2 protocols have additional treatments that are a part of the overall protocol. These are treatments that enhance the main objective, destroying the cancer cells, stimulating the immune system and eliminating toxins.

...Cellect...

One of the main components of this protocol is a nutritional powder called Cellect. It has excellent results with nearly all cancers and other chronic or terminal health issues. The formula was developed by a Pre-Med/Bio Chemist named Fred Eichorn who cured himself of pancreatic cancer.

Fortunately, there is expert advice and support in the application of this protocol. Mike Vrentas has well over 10 years experience in alternative medicine and is the designer of this protocol. Mike provides detailed CD's with information on this protocol and very reasonable telephone support if needed.

The first part of the protocol involves ordering the Cellect powder. The product is marketed as Maxi-Blend. They have flavored and unflavored. The unflavored is recommended because the flavored requires taking a larger amount due to the added flavorings.

The patient would start out with ½ to 1 scoop a day and see how well it is tolerated. The recommended dosage calls for 4 scoops a day. Very ill patients may have to work their way up to that amount. There are occasionally problems with constipation so Cod Liver Oil capsules are included with the product. Again, monitor the consistency of your bowel movements while taking the Cellect, if they become too loose, reduce the dosage of the cod liver capsules.

There are alternative medical practitioners that sell the Cellect under the brand name "Trican" which would increase the cost a bit so purchasing the product from http://www.cellect.org/ under the name Maxi-Blend should save you some money.

The treatment with the Cellect calls for 4 scoops daily which times 7 days would equal 1 container. The Cellect also comes in capsules but the dosage requires taking 24 capsules so the powder would be much easier to administer.

The powder contains Calcium, Magnesium, Zinc, Shark Cartilage, Milk Thistle, Chromium Piccolinate, Vitamin E, Colostrum, Selenium, Lecithin, 74 Trace Minerals and Gelatin, (7g serving). It is recommended to space the servings throughout the day and to not take the Cellect on an empty stomach.

The Cod Liver capsules are included with the powder. The cost of the Cellect (Maxi-Blend) product for a 1 week supply is $100.00 as of this writing.

The main reason for taking the Cellect/Maxi-Blend product is to buy time for the cancer patient. It is a highly recommended nutritional supplement to support non-cancerous cells. The Cellect helps to revive non-cancerous cells, giving the treatment of choice much more time to start working and effect the cancerous cells. For late stage cancers buying extra time is crucial.

Even if you do not decide to use the full Cellect-Budwig protocol it is still one of the highest rated nutritional supplements to support normal, healthy cells. Cellect should not be used with any therapy that reduces ATP energy production as the Cellect raises ATP (adenosine triphosphate). Cellect should not be used with the Protocel Protocol or The Amazon Factor Protocol. Whichever protocol you decide upon, the vendor and or adviser to that particular protocol will recommend any additional supplementation.

Cellect should also not be used if you are taking Hydrazine Sulphate. For the majority of any of the other protocols Cellect is not only one of your best choices for nutritional support, but is considered mandatory for late stage cancer patients.

If a late stage cancer patient is unable to eat and is being fed through a feeding tube, there is a liquid mineral supplement available. The supplement is called "Live" and is made by the Nuriche company.

...Budwig Protocol/Flaxseed Oil & Cottage Cheese...

The second part of the protocol is the Budwig diet. The Budwig diet is the Flaxseed Oil and Cottage Cheese diet. I have an extensive article and chapter on the benefits of the Flaxseed Oil and Cottage diet protocol in this book. Please refer to that chapter for all the details.

...High Radio Frequency Generator...

The third part of this protocol is a High Radio Frequency Generator and a Plasma Ray Tube Amplifier. The addition and combination of this therapy has proven to be very powerful. This High RF Generator with Plasma Amplifier is an electromedicine device modeled after Royal Rife's original designs.

The majority of the electromedicine devices are very gentle and many times the patient doesn't even know they are receiving a treatment. The addition of this device with the Cellect-Budwig protocol is that it helps to quickly and safely rid the body of cancerous cells. It can also very effectively reduce pain.

The highlight and greatest benefit of the High RF electromedicine device is that it reverts cancerous cells into normal cells. This is different from the majority of the other therapies where the body has to deal with dead and dying microbial debris.

This technology is based on the protocols of Royal Rife, the subject of the previous chapter. There are many companies out there selling "Rife Machines," whether or not they comply with his original specifications and designs is unknown.

According to the ICRF (Independent Cancer Research Foundation) and Webster Kehr, an alternative cancer researcher, author and webmaster of cancertutor.com, nothing compares to the High RF Generator & Plasma Amplifier which can be purchased here http://www.frequencystore.com/.

This device acts like a radio tower, it broadcasts a signal that travels more than 50 meters. Because of this you can utilize it on any type of cancer, including some of the more difficult cancers to treat like brain cancer, bone cancer, pancreatic cancer, colon cancer, liver cancer, lymphoma's and leukemia.

The cost of the High RF Generator with the plasma amplifier costs around $4,800. For those who cannot afford the more expensive amplifier there is a less expensive amplifier called a linear amplifier. This amplifier uses electrodes, whereas the plasma amplifier does not require electrodes. It broadcasts similar to a radio tower through the use of an antenna. The cost of the High RF Generator with the linear amplifier costs about $2,500. A considerable difference in cost but not nearly as powerful as the plasma amplifier.

The other benefit of the plasma amplifier is that it directly reaches all parts of the body. That would be the difference between radio waves and electrical current emanating from the electrodes.

There is a "*Warning*" with electromedicine protocols. They cannot be used at the same time as strong prescription medications. Because of the way electromedicine works by reaching inside of the cells, it may allow these prescription drugs to get inside of the cells. The majority of prescription drugs were not designed to permeate the interior of the cell. This can pose a serious problem if they are powerful drugs. Time released prescription drugs should be taken 1 hour after the electromedicine protocol is finished for the day.

You can go to this website to find out more about the High RF (Radio Frequency) Generator and Plasma Amplifier. http://www.frequencystore.com/_to visit the site.

...Laetrile/Vitamin B17...

The 4th part of this protocol is Vitamin B17 or Laetrile. Laetrile has been used in the treatment of cancer for decades. In fact it was a part of the IV treatments my first wife was receiving along with the IV Vitamin C therapy. It was shortly into her remarkable progress that the FDA mysteriously removed it from the market.

It was in 1950 that a very dedicated biochemist by the name of Ernest T. Krebs isolated a new vitamin that he specifically numbered B17 and named Laetrile. It was believed by many that Dr. Krebs had finally found the key to controlling all cancers.

This was met with extreme prejudice by the exorbitantly powerful pharmaceutical conglomerate and they proceeded to launch a massive propaganda campaign against its efficacy and use.

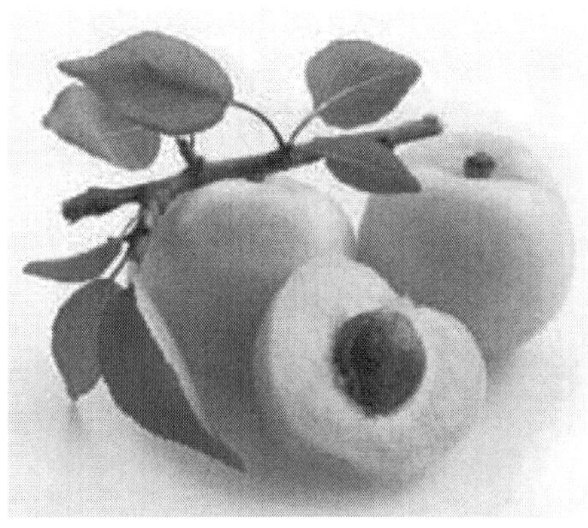

Even today, Laetrile is touted to be a complete fraud and pure quackery by the medical establishment, even though thousands of patients every year travel to Mexico and other countries to obtain the healing effects of Laetrile. The overwhelming success stories speak for themselves. Many late stage cancer patients are alive today because of Laetrile.

The following story is from a testimonial on the use of Laetrile. This patient was diagnosed with cancer of the colon which had metastasized to the bladder. He was then scheduled for surgery. During the operation, the surgeons found the cancer so widespread that it was impossible to remove it all. They cleared his blockage by severing the colon and performed a colonostomy.

Several months later, this patient was informed that the cancer had worsened and spread. He was told he only had a few months to live. This man was a registered nurse and had heard of the successes using Laetrile. He was more or less out of options from conventional medicine so he decided to give Laetrile a try.

After 6 months of treatment with Laetrile, this man totally surprised his doctors by feeling well enough to resume most of his normal routines at work. An exploratory examination of the bladder revealed that the cancer was gone. He then asked his doctors if there was anyway to put his colon back together again. He was then again scheduled for surgery.

During surgery they found him to be, much to their amazement, totally cancer free. They decided to proceed, and successfully reconnected his colon. This was a rare and first time procedure for this hospital. He is alive and well and continues to be cancer free. Oops, that's not supposed to happen if you listen to the mainstream medical propaganda.

Ok, 1 more testimonial just because it is so inspiring and especially because this treatment is clouded in such an aura of deception. This particular gentlemen was diagnosed with Lymphocytic Leukemia plus cancer of the spleen and liver. Even though his spleen was removed, he was informed he only had a few more months to live and even that was pushing the proverbial envelope.

They suggested he do chemotherapy, not for a cure, but to possibly buy a few more weeks. He decided not to buy. This gentlemen refused and decided he would try the Laetrile. The doctor who administered the Laetrile informed him how and why Laetrile was working. He then suggested intravenous shots of 30 cc's daily for the next 3 weeks. The Dr. also recommended enzymes, food supplements and a cancer diet.

It only took a few days before he started feeling better. Unfortunately, on his 3rd visit to the doctor, he regretfully informed him that he could no longer administer the Laetrile. He was being threatened with having his medical license revoked if he continued administering the Laetrile. The Dr. ended up showing this man's wife how to administer the Laetrile. The Dr. sold them what he had and gave them the information of where they could obtain more.

This man continued the treatments and was progressively feeling better every day. He then got a call from his original doctor asking why he had not returned for his chemotherapy treatments. This doctor informed him he was playing a risky and very dangerous game with his life. He finally persuaded him to return for the chemotherapy treatments. The side effects were horrendous, his eyes burned and his stomach was on fire. It had only been a few days and he was so weak he could hardly get out of bed. He felt that the treatment would kill him far before the actual cancer would.

He decided to stop the chemotherapy treatments altogether and return to the Laetrile, diet and food supplements. In a very short time he started feeling better, even though he was now battling two afflictions, the leftover chemotherapy residuals and the cancer.

As time passed he found himself able to resume his exercise routines without tiring. He is now 75 years of age and 20 years beyond their prediction of only a few more months to live. He continues to play racquetball twice a week.

Ironically, after this gentleman had successfully defeated his cancer, he was approached by a doctor one day. This was a medical doctor that was currently prescribing chemotherapy at a well known hospital.

Unfortunately, this doctor's wife was extremely ill with cancer and he wanted to know the details of how this gentleman had defeated his cancer unconventionally. The gentleman then asked the doctor why he didn't just prescribe the chemotherapy for his wife. The doctor replied that he would never give chemotherapy to any of his family members or his friends. Apparently this was not an isolated incident, other doctors came to this gentleman with the same question.

The majority of patients using Laetrile report very positive responses. They report a noticeable increase in their overall well being and outlook on life. Along with hope, they report an increased appetite, weight gain, a discernible reduction or elimination of pain and a more healthful color to their skin. Thousands of cases have reported a complete and total regression of all cancer signs and symptoms.

Vitamin B17 or Laetrile is also known as "Amygdalin" and is commonly found online under the name Amygdalin. A medical doctor from the U.S. FDA once stated that Laetrile contains "Free" Hydrogen Cyanide which is toxic. In fact, I'm sure you have heard the story from someone that apricot seeds and apple seeds contain cyanide and are dangerous and toxic to our health. "Free" hydrogen cyanide is a whole different apple altogether, pun intended. The truth being that there is no "free" hydrogen cyanide in Laetrile.

Laetrile does contain the cyanide radical. This same cyanide radical is in Vitamin B12, blackberries, blueberries and strawberries.

There is a huge difference in "free" hydrogen cyanide and the cyanide radical, they are 2 completely different compounds. Similar to something like pure sodium (Na+) - one of the most toxic substances known to mankind and sodium chloride (NaCl) - which is table salt, again 2 totally different compounds. Please don't buy this convenient story they are trying to sell.

It's funny how the conventional medical authorities lay in wait for those patients that still die after receiving Laetrile treatments. This way they can scream from the rooftops "See, Laetrile is a fraud!"

Laetrile very safely and effectively kills cancer cells without the accumulation of dangerous toxic debris. Mainly because it does not kill the cancer cells too quickly. IV therapy is the most effective way to administer Laetrile but, unfortunately, the FDA has now made this illegal in the U.S.

Another potent method of ingesting B17 (Laetrile) is by eating apricot kernels. Apricot kernels are rich in Vitamin B17. Laetrile tablets are also available online where they will ship to you direct. The tablets are typically 500mg. Apricot kernels are a more effective way for your body to utilize the Laetrile as you get the benefit of the whole. Meaning you receive the Laetrile the way Mother Nature packaged it. You receive its benefits along with all the other co-factors of the whole package, increasing the body's ability to more effectively assimilate and utilize the Laetrile.

I've said it before that man cannot compete with God's original packaging. Anything you put into your body, be it vitamins, minerals or any other type of supplement, needs to be packaged as close to God's original composition as possible. That way you take advantage of all the micro-nutrients and other trace elements. They were put there for the purpose of a synergistic and complete, everything working to assist and aid each other, complex. It's a team effort. You can't pick out the best player in the game and play a game of baseball. Man cannot create a superior form. Deal with it. A billion of the brightest minds in science and medicine cannot compare to the extreme, over the top, indescribable brilliance of our Creator God. We are still trying to figure out the incomprehensible architecture of His creation, us.

As usual, the amount of Laetrile needed for your particular cancer will differ according to how far advanced your cancer is. In a statement by Ernest T. Krebs Jr. he states that if you have cancer, the single most important issue would be to get the maximum amount of Vitamin B17 into your body in the shortest amount of time. This is secondary to the medical skill involved in administering it, which Dr. Krebs believes to be relatively minimal.

There are numerous vendors of apricot kernels on the internet. This is the most potent way to administer Laetrile besides IV liquid injections. In the middle of the apricot is a hard shell. If you break open the hard shell with a hammer or a nutcracker there is a small seed or kernel inside, kind of looks like an almond. It is actually much softer than an almond. This is what is rich in Vitamin B17 or Laetrile. A word of warning, they are really bitter. Just get it over with and think of all the wonderful things this Laetrile will do for your body.

As I mentioned before with other supplements it is best to gradually build up to a therapeutic dose of Laetrile. Many start with 3-6 apricot seeds a day and slowly work up to between 20-30 per day. Vitamin C complements Laetrile. The 2 taken together, in large doses, are a cancer treatment in themselves. Like I said before, my wife was having remarkable success with the intravenous application of the vitamin C/Laetrile combination.

Regardless if you have cancer or not, I highly recommend adding apricot kernels to your daily health regimen. Start with 3 and work your way up to 7-10. It is definitely an acquired taste. Find something to mix it with or just chase it down immediately with something flavorful, orange juice works great. You'll get used to it. Focus on the benefits. Some people even like the taste. Maybe it's just me, maybe not, you need to find out for yourself.

...Juicing...

The 5th part of this protocol involves juicing. The benefits of juicing have been described in other chapters. Generally, building up to 40-50 ounces of freshly made juice a day for adults is required.

Make sure to space them out during the day and gradually work your way up to that amount.

One of the best juices you can make is carrot/apple juice. With carrot juicing being a treatment in itself along with a few other complementary supplements. Carrots should be a large part of your juicing protocol. If you decide to use an apple with your carrot juice, use the whole apple, seeds and all. Carrots have a very powerful anti-cancer component. For more information on an English gentleman that cured his cancer, you can check into Jason Winter's. He drank several glasses of carrot juice daily. He also makes a delicious tea he simply calls Jason Winter's Tea. It is an herbal anti-cancer tea and is very good. I used that also with my wife.

...Detoxification...

The 6th part of this protocol is the importance of detoxification. All of these aspects of the Cellect-Budwig Protocol are discussed in the audio cd's from the website along with step by step instructions.

...Sunshine...

The 7th and final aspect of this protocol is the need to spend some quality time out in the sunshine. This you should also start gradually, especially if you are not used to being out in the sun. Starting at about 15-20 minutes a day and working your way up to about 40-45 minutes a day. Believe it or not a good majority of sunscreens can cause skin cancer, big surprise, so remember not to use sunscreen.

Warning: Do not attempt this protocol alone. It's really important to have some sort of expert or medically trained professional to consult with. You should let your doctor know what you are doing. Many will dismiss you as a lunatic or advise you that you are risking your life but the statistics and success stories speak for themselves.

Mike Vrentas, who designed this protocol has an audio series of CD's that run about 5 ½ hours. It is critical that you listen to these. The CD's are the result of many hours consulting and speaking with many different cancer patients that have utilized the protocol.

Because of the many potential, unexpected symptoms associated with this or any protocol, the audio CD's are a mandatory requirement. It just makes sense to arm yourself with any and all aspects of the program. In fact it wouldn't hurt to listen to them more than once. Listen once, start the protocol, then listen again as whoever is being treated progresses.

Even if you decide this is not the treatment you want to pursue you will still gain immense benefit from the information. You can go to his website http://www.cellectbudwig.com/ and download them immediately or order them on CD. The cost is under $50 dollars.

Mike provides in the audio series, information he obtained from many individual cases and he also includes the science behind the protocol. He includes information for you to better understand why and how the protocol works. How it re-balances and rebuilds your internal body chemistry. He also goes over details on how to deal with detoxification issue's and side effects.

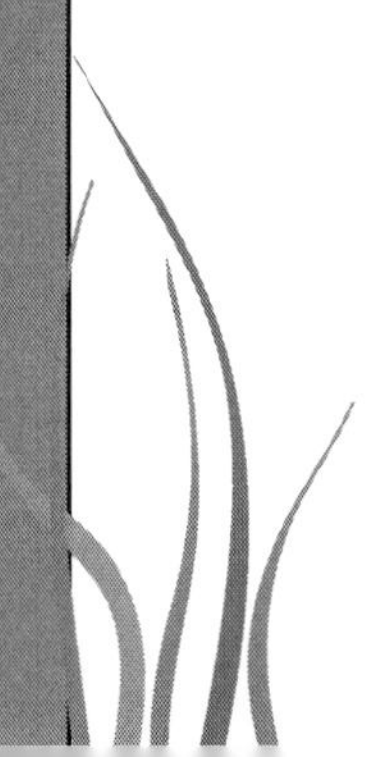

Chapter 14

Bob Beck Protocol

The Bob Beck Protocol is one of the most effective, immune boosting protocols available. This Protocol works by destroying microbes within the body and the blood thereby supercharging the immune system to more effectively and efficiently destroy cancer and other evil, uninvited, invading organisms.

It's pretty obvious that our overly polluted bodies have destroyed the power and functionality of our immune systems, our main-line of defense. We are slowly but surely slipping further and further into a life of ever increasing infirmities and disease. Why? Our immune systems are stagnant, ineffective, unbalanced, filthy, clogged up and downright exhausted.

Dr. Beck was searching for a way to lighten the load on the immune system and clean up the mess, you know, sweep the floor and clear the clutter that was inhibiting its ability to be effective. This would enable the body to take care of itself via its own, innate and ultimately supreme, mechanism of defense. A fully functioning, supercharged and well balanced immune system.

This is a very important aspect of the Bob Beck Protocol. This protocol succeeds by strengthening the immune system. This treatment does not kill cancer cells directly. It clears, cleans and supercharges the blood to a point where the immune system is able to work again and perform its ultimate role in the body.

It is based on the science that disease and or cancer cannot survive with a well functioning, peak performing immune system. Our bodies are not capable of harboring disease. Disease became part of our biology thru improper foods, tainted water and polluted air.

Our bodies, when fresh off the assembly line, before the introduction of toxic influence, were perfectly suited to fend off any and all foreign entities.

No doubt Dr. Beck was inspired and motivated by the earlier experiments and successes of William Lyman, Steven Kaali and most would agree, the originator of this technology, Dr. Royal Rife. Unfortunately, Royal Rife's research was pretty much destroyed and forever, or so it seemed, buried beyond recovery. Dr. Beck was determined to bring this method of attack back into the realm of possibilities.

Dr. Beck, being a well acclaimed and award winning physicist, put his own genius spin on some of the earlier studies and developed a gentle and effective way people could apply these simple protocols at home.

There are 4 parts to his protocol. The first 2 are based on micro-current therapy for cleansing the blood. Research from highly respected universities along with the experiments of William Lyman and Steven Kaali confirm these findings, that microbes, pathogens, viruses, bacteria, fungi and parasites can be eliminated through the use of micro-currents or electrification.

Warning: The Bob Beck Protocol should not be the treatment of choice for advanced, fast growing and late stage cancers. It is an excellent cancer therapy although it works on the concept of super charging the immune system which can take some time.

Since the Bob Beck Protocol supercharges the immune system it is not only just a cancer treatment. It will help, by way of the supercharged immune system, any type of affliction you may be experiencing. Starting with one of the more direct cancer/ microbe killing protocols would be advised and then introducing the Bob Beck Protocol. If you are dealing with a less aggressive type of cancer than this is a highly effective treatment and can be utilized for the rest of your life.

Also, chemotherapy and or other powerful drugs cannot be used with this protocol as it creates electroporation. Electroporation is the phenomena which can potentially allow the drugs to find their way inside of the cell.

...Blood Electrification...

The first part of the protocol consists of placing an electrode over the main 2 arteries in the wrist. The Ulnar and the Radial. These electrodes are then connected to a small device that sends out a DC electrical charge, somewhere between 50-100 micro-amps. Dr. Beck suggests carefully marking the exact location of the arteries on the wrists. Use a visible marker to make sure the electrodes are placed and aligned properly over these 2 arteries.

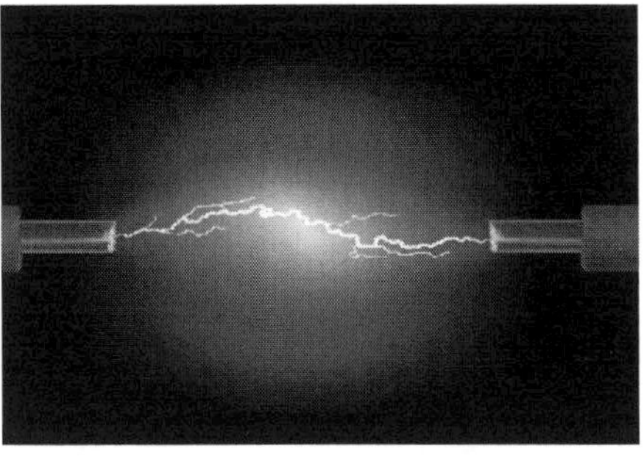

This very slight electrical charge increases ATP (Adenosine Triphosphate) activity within the mitochrondia of the cell, thus increasing the cells energy production. This increased energy production increases the beneficial activity and efficiency of the cell, strengthening the cells effectiveness.

The electrodes are held in place by a velcro fastened wristband. The electrification unit is also attached to the upper arm via a velcro fastened strap. It is a small, lightweight unit and operates on a 9 volt DC electrical current. It can be worn while performing other daily tasks or chores.

It is typically used for 2 hours a day. Many people start at 20 minutes for the first few days and gradually increase up to the 2 hour target level. It's the same with any of the therapies, if you have the luxury of starting slowly than that is usually the best strategy.

The electrical charge emitted by this device is very slight. It produces a very light but constant tingling sensation. Don't be frightened by the thought of a constant electrical charge being overly annoying and not being able to deal with it. Patients have described it as a light tickling or tingling sensation. It is a very subtle amount and you will quite rapidly and very easily become accustomed to it's application.

Dr. Beck became involved in this type of therapy after reading an article in Science News Magazine that had been published back in 1991. It was an article from the Albert Einstein College of Medicine where they had inadvertently found a cure for AIDS.

This Earth shattering information was presented at the first international symposium on combination therapies in Washington D.C. Unfortunately, any trace of the information and or documentation was nowhere to be found. Dr. Beck hired a private investigator who eventually was able to obtain a copy from an attendee at the conference where it was originally introduced.

Dr. Beck tells the story of an ironic and funny thing happening 2 years later when the patent just happened by chance to pop up. Don't you just love it when things like that materialize?

The U.S. Government Patent Office described in detail, through the contents of the patent, the entire process. It went on to say how the protocol would attenuate any bacteria or virus, (including HIV/AIDS), parasites and all fungi within the bloodstream. The best part being that the process was completely harmless to any healthy, normal cells.

By attenuate, it means that this electrification process would diminish or weaken the outer protein layer of the microbe. In this weakened state the microbe is unable to replicate or breed and simply dies off.

I'm sure you are again wondering why the entire world doesn't know about this, right? A cure for HIV/AIDS. Hmmmm, seems it kind of got swept under the Persian rug. It would appear to be business as usual for the infirmity establishment.

...Magnetic Pulser...

Anyway, back to the Beck Protocol. So, the first part of the protocol is the blood electrification procedure. The second part would be the magnetic pulser. The magnetic pulser helps to dislodge microbes and any other bacteria that are not currently in the bloodstream. This is more or less the clean up crew. Whatever microbes were not affected with the blood electrification process are dislodged from elsewhere in the body with a magnetic pulse.

These would be the microbes hiding out in the tissues, the lymphatic system, the digestive system, root canals and so on. The magnetic pulser would entice them out of their cozy little hideaways and allow them to enter the bloodstream where they would end up being disabled by the blood electrification process. Many patients utilize the magnetic pulser prior to the blood electrification process. That way, additional microbes find their way into the blood.

The magnetic pulser is extremely easy to use. It consists of the base unit and a handheld paddle. The magnetic pulser is capable of penetrating up to 9+ inches into the body and easily passes this charge through tissue and through bone. It is completely painless and quiet.

The magnetic Pulser typically runs in 20 minute cycles or a little over 200 pulses. It then needs to be turned off for around the same amount of time to allow for cool down. It will send out a pulse every few seconds. You simply place the paddle around various parts of the body and pulse several times.

You will have to remove any metal jewelry, watches, metal belt buckles or anything else metal on your body. Keep it away from your mouth if you have any metal fillings. If you do have metal fillings they need to be removed anyway. Just don't use the magnetic pulser to remove them. You will also want to keep it away from other metal or electronic appliances. The magnetic pulser also cannot be used on patients with a pacemaker.

Since the magnetic pulser breaks away microbes from areas other than the blood, it will help to clear and open up stagnant or constricted lymphatic pathways. It would be beneficial to find a detailed schematic of the lymphatic system and target the major lymph nodes of the body with the magnetic pulser.

Other areas that should be targeted are the organs, digestive areas and any parts of the body that may be congested or inflamed. Tumors and or other cancerous areas should also be on the schedule of targeted magnetic pulsing.

The effectiveness of pulsed magnetic fields has been well documented. The research confirms its effectiveness in improving circulation through the blood and through the lymphatic system. It also accelerated tissue regeneration, reduced inflammation, helped in regulating nervous system disorders and was helpful in alleviating and reducing pain.

Studies across the U.S. have verified the claim that the use of magnetic pulsing increases the rate of healing in fractures of the bone. It also helps to initiate healing in stubborn breaks and fractures that had previously been unable to progress.

Pulsed magnetic fields increase oxygen respiration at the cellular level, greatly improving the efficiency of cell metabolism, and enhancing mineral absorption and exchange. From these increased benefits and improvements in helping to strengthen the capacity of the immune system, patients have been able to overcome heart, lung and gastrointestinal issues too. Patients have also reported improvements in overcoming infections, skin diseases and rheumatism.

...Colloidal Silver...

The third part of the protocol involves colloidal silver and its amazing benefits to the body. It is a completely safe, bio-available, non-toxic, non-carcinogenic, non-accumulative, all natural antibiotic.

Colloidal Silver is an old fashioned, albeit very powerful, sterilizing, purifying, unadulterated, odorless, liquid medicine. It is antimicrobial and effectively kills bacteria, molds, viruses, parasites and fungi.

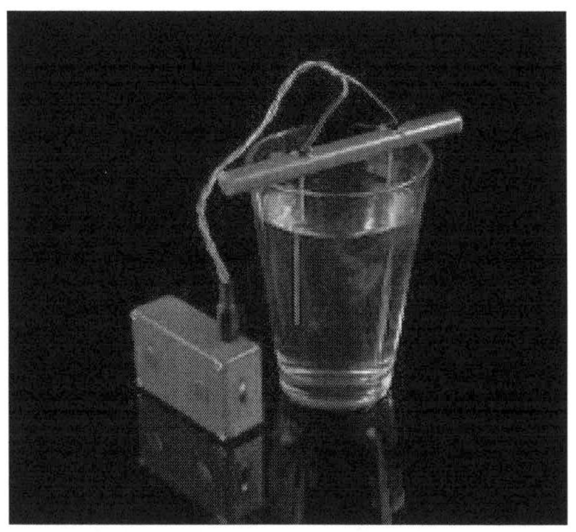

Colloidal Silver is an electrically charged, micro cluster of fine silver particles suspended in distilled water. It is completely safe taken internally or externally. Colloidal Silver may be administered sublingually, intravenously, vaginally, rectally, topically, orally and intramuscularly. It may also be used as eye drops for infections such as pink eye and as an effective ear tonic.

It can be added to a vaporizer or humidifier and may also be atomized and used for nasal or lung inhalation. It should not be used with humidifiers that boil the water, it should only be used with ultrasonic humidifiers.

Colloidal Silver is non-accumulative in the body. The silver is removed by the liver and somewhere around 90% of that is eliminated in the bile through the large intestine. The remainder is eliminated in the urine.

The power of colloidal silver and its ability to destroy microbes is well established. The Soviets add silver to sterilize their recycled water in the space station. Japanese companies use silver to purify air and also as an additive for disinfecting foods. Some Japanese clothing companies sew in a piece of silver thread into their clothing to protect from ultraviolet radiation.

The uses and benefits of colloidal silver are seemingly endless. It has been used to treat brain disorders, reproductive disorders, circulation problems, headaches, joint pain, sinus problems, acne and the list goes on and on.

The amount needed for your particular situation will vary according to the quality of the colloidal silver and the parts per million in suspension. Applied kineseology is a very accurate way of determining the amount needed for your present condition.

It can also be used safely on your pets. You can safely add around a teaspoon to their drinking water depending on the size of your pet and the size of your water bowl. A teaspoon would be the average for a medium sized dog. The best part being that you need not be afraid of overdosing. If anything you might notice a loose stool. If this happens, you can just adjust the dose down a bit and monitor.

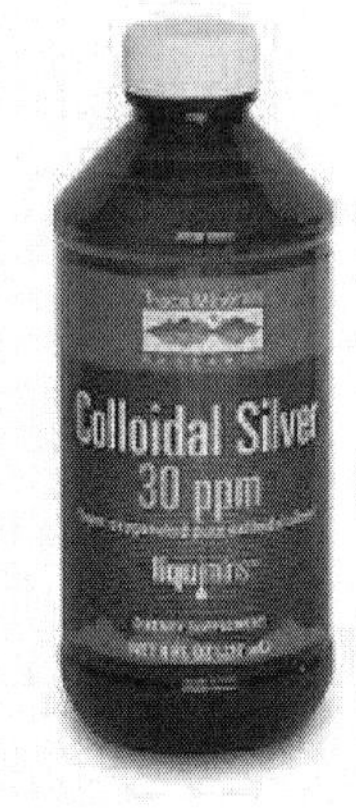

Some cities around the world use silver to sterilize their public drinking water supply. It is used extensively on burn victims because of its ability to advance healing and regeneration. Many hospitals use silver coated urinary catheters to reduce the incidence of infection.

It has also proven to be effective against the SARS virus, AIDS, anthrax, typhoid, influenza, whooping cough, diphtheria and the common cold. Silver is very effective against malaria where it is distributed by volunteers who very courageously track deep into remote jungle locations around the world to deliver it.

Properly administered and properly brewed, high quality colloidal silver will not cause argyria (turn your skin blue), although that is a very well known, well publicized, mis-information campaign used to dissuade people from using it in place of their beloved anti-psychotics, oops I mean antibiotics.

The FDA at one point claimed it killed over 650 different disease causing pathogens. Colloidal silver is a positive charged, bio-electric mineral that binds to negatively charged free radicals and or pathogens. It interrupts the biological function of the pathogen, destroying its ability to reproduce. The best part being that organisms cannot build up a tolerance or resistance to it like antibiotics.

Numerous studies have been done on Colloidal Silver at universities like UCLA, USC, Harvard, Columbia, Loyola, UC Berkeley, Brigham Young, Alabama, Arizona, Syracuse and Yale. No one has ever overdosed on Colloidal Silver and it is completely harmless to humans.

Prior to the inception of antibiotics, colloidal silver and its curative powers had been known for hundreds of years. A Dr. Ron Surowitz, an Osteopath and head of the Florida Osteopathic Medical Association stated that the use of antibiotics almost always necessitates the use of colloidal silver to get rid of the fungus and yeast caused by the antibiotic.

Yeh right, how many times has your doctor informed you that the antibiotic you are using has the potential to totally disrupt your immune system, destroy valuable, beneficial bacteria, and manifest the growth of harmful yeast and fungal infections? Then, of course tell you that you should use colloidal silver afterwords to clean up the devastation left by the antibiotic. Does never ring a bell? That's what I thought.

Ok, everybody knows that silver is a precious metal and a great looking piece of jewelry but, many do not realize or know that silver is a trace mineral essential to the body. This all goes back to our overly depleted soils and our obvious lack of this essential mineral.

A Dr. Robert O. Becker, a prominent and well recognized figure in electro-medical and cellular regeneration technologies stated that, a silver deficiency is responsible for an unbalanced and malfunctioning immune system. He concluded that there was a very close correlation between low silver levels in the body and sickness.

Ingesting silver in colloidal form allows instant permeability into our cells and tissues. As I have said before, without minerals, vitamins are very poorly utilized by the body if at all. Scientific research confirms the interrelationship and synergistic qualities that exist between vitamins and minerals.

It has been affirmed more than once or twice, that the single leading cause of death in the U.S. is malnutrition. Of course malnutrition is never listed on the death certificate nor is the headline in any public media correspondence but, if whatever is listed was investigated, like a murder is likely to be, and trailed back to the primary cause and killer of the host, not surprisingly, it would be pre-meditated malnutrition.

Our depleted and sadly inadequate man-made soils have taken a huge bite out of our immunity. The abundance of all known, natural mineral elements, like silver, present in our food and water are the secret and synergistic harmonies necessary for all living matter.

It is truly magical how a substance measured in parts per million can have such a profound effect on the human body.

...Ozonated Water...

This is the 4th part of the Bob Beck protocol. It involves the use of an ozone water generator to purify water in your home. This is a protocol that can and should be used in combination with the other therapies.

This is another way of rapidly adding oxygen to the body and bloodstream. It is also an immune system stimulator. Ozone benefits the detoxification process by enhancing the bodies ability to rid itself of dead and dying toxic debris initiated by the blood electrification protocol and magnetic pulser.

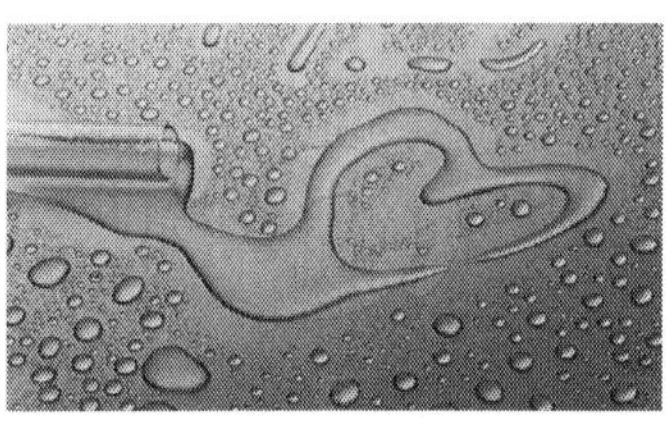

Ozonating your water will kill any E.coli, yeast, cysts, salmonella, listeria, bacteria, microbes and other viruses that may be present in your water source. Ozonated water binds singlet molecules of oxygen together. This binding is very unstable as the singlet molecules are constantly breaking free. This is a good thing as the extra singlet oxygen molecules will seek out and bind to free radicals and toxins in the body.

These extra oxygen molecules help to oxidize and eliminate impurities from the bloodstream. It also heightens cognitive functions in the brain by increasing oxygen saturation throughout.

You can even bathe in ozonated water. It is considered by most a very energizing experience. The ozonated, oxygen charged water is absorbed by the skin and is another way of quickly oxygenating the body. Since the ozone is so unstable it constantly jumps on the surface of the water, if this creates a problem you can open a window or set up a fan to help quiet the reaction.

Water ozonators are also used to purify and cleanse foodstuffs. It will destroy any germs or other micro-organisms and actually extend the shelf life of your fruits, vegetables or whatever else you decide to ozonate.

When you ozonate your water you have to drink it immediately. The ozone in the water will turn back into oxygen fully, in about a half an hour. Give the glass a swirl before you drink it as the ozone will rise to the top. The oxygen atoms are very unstable, highly energized and quickly break down.

Whatever protocol you decide upon, an ozone water and food purifier would be a great benefit. An ozone air purifier would also be a great benefit to your healing. As far as I know it is a fairly recent addition and is being utilized with the Gerson Therapy with very favorable results

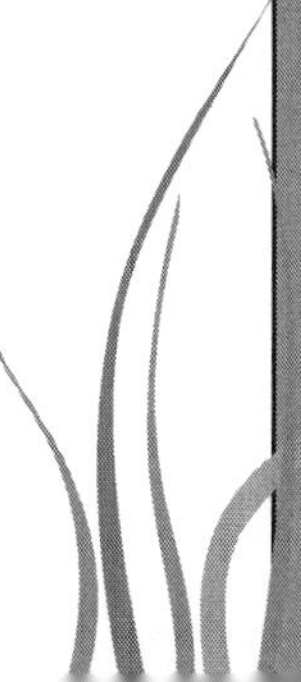

Chapter 15

Cesium Chloride Protocol

This is yet another extremely effective treatment for early and late stage cancer patients. It is a very strong and powerful treatment dealing once again with the pH of the body. This protocol works by effectively and rapidly alkalizing the cancer cell.

If you remember earlier in the book, cancer cannot survive in an alkaline environment. It thrives in an acidic environment. Because of Cesium Chlorides ability to manifest rapid results, it is highly recommended to have support, advice and or guidance from a well informed, well educated vendor of ionic cesium chloride or, a well educated, alternative, holistic medicine practitioner familiar with its application.

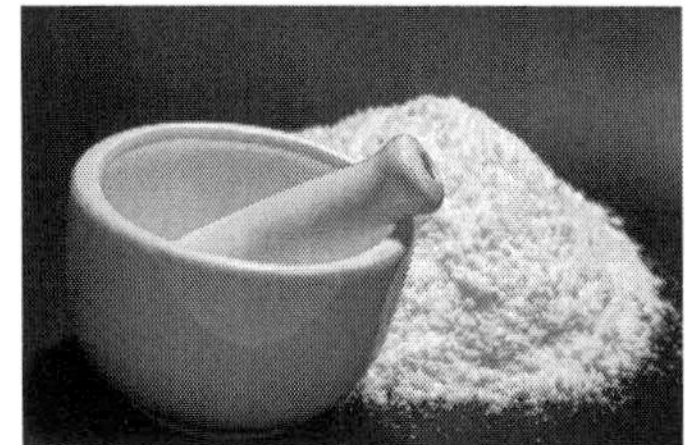

Cesium chloride as an alternative cancer treatment has been around since the 1980's. Back then, the treatment consisted of a powdered form of Cesium Chloride, typically administered in capsule form. It is now much more effective and much more readily assimilated and absorbed in an ionic, liquid mineral form.

Cesium chloride is Nature's most alkaline mineral. One of the benefits of liquid, ionic minerals like Cesium Chloride is that it will typically not build up to a toxic level in the body. If by chance this does occur, there are certain signs and symptoms to look out for.

Typically, when you have reached your limit, you may experience a pins and needles feeling in your fingertips or they can become very tender to the touch, your feet may feel unusually cold, turn purple and you may experience a feeling similar to frostbite in your feet.

This just re-enforces the need for experienced guidance during your treatment. Any treatment needs to be approached with reasoning, wisdom and logic. Remember the saying "For every action, there is an equal and opposite reaction." Pay close attention to any reactions. Believe me, the reactions and or side effects from natural treatments pale in comparison to the side effects experienced with conventional, allopathic treatments.

Another reason for guidance and support while using Cesium Chloride is the need for certain supplementation while on the therapy. There is strong evidence that Laetrile greatly enhances the cells ability to utilize the cesium chloride maybe even better than the vitamins typically recommended during treatment. Those vitamins include; vitamin C, vitamin A, zinc, selenium, magnesium and calcium.

As always, the more of these vitamins and minerals you can get from eating whole, organic foods the better. When you take them in whole form, as I have mentioned before, your body receives the other micro-nutrients and co-factors associated with it and your body is able to utilize it far more effectively than an isolated version. There truly is no comparison.

Research supports the use of 6 grams per day of cesium chloride. Usually 2 grams, 3 times per day. At this amount they have determined it to have a zero toxic effect. Of course the amount you need will be affected by your own personal state and or current condition. That determination is best left to an experienced professional.

High doses of Cesium Chloride for cancer treatment leaches potassium from the body. It does this by drawing potassium into the cell, so, taking a liquid, ionic potassium supplement is strongly advised and more or less mandatory. In other words, it needs to be part of the protocol.

Potassium deficiency can lead to heart attacks and even death so, it is not something to take lightly or overlook. The ratio of potassium to cesium is normally 3 to 1 but can be adjusted up to as high as 6 to 1 for those that may already have a compromised or weakened heart condition.

What actually happens is, as the body becomes more alkaline, this movement of potassium into the cells leads to a deficiency of serum potassium in the body.

Finding a health professional willing to monitor your progress and your potential deficiency levels would be greatly beneficial and highly advised. They would be able to check for any imbalances or deficiencies that need to be adjusted while on the protocol.

This is a very critical component to the protocol. Low serum potassium levels creates a condition called Hypokalemia. High serum potassium levels creates a condition called hyperkalemia. It may sound strange but the majority of potassium, around 98%, is found within the cells. It is typically a very small percentage that circulates in the blood, serum potassium.

It plays a crucial role in the body. It helps regulate the action of the heart and the pathways linking the brain and the muscles. Excess potassium is normally excreted by the kidneys. Hyperkalemia is typically caused by obstructed or insufficient kidney function.

The symptoms of low and high serum potassium levels are very similar. Muscle weakness, irregular heart rhythms and fatigue. These are very serious conditions and can be fatal. This information is not meant to frighten you from considering the treatment, it's just to make sure you have all your ducks lined up.

All self administered, alternative treatments need your full attention to every possible detail and or symptom. You just need to understand and know your body. I'm sure this is a whole new world for the majority of you.

Monitoring and testing your potassium, magnesium, calcium, uric acid, electrolytes and sodium levels every 2-4 weeks is recommended. Keep track of any symptoms or spikes in your blood pressure or heart rate. You can certainly do this yourself. This should be done regardless of what treatment you decide upon.

The vast majority of the protocols in alternative medicine require the patients involvement in their own recovery. Whether it is you or you have the benefit of a caregiver or spouse, you are your own best detective and self-taught, stay at home doctor.

Changing your diet and lifestyle are crucial to your recovery and the effectiveness of any of the treatments. The same is true for the cesium chloride therapy. Switching to a high alkaline diet rich in raw fruits and vegetables is a must.

Because of cesium chlorides high alkalinity, taking it on an empty stomach can cause intestinal upset. It can cause nausea as it will react with the acids in the stomach. It is best taken after a meal to avoid any potential issue's. The ionic cesium chloride and the ionic potassium should not be taken together, usually about an hour apart is best.

Remember, depending on the severity of your condition and the amount of cesium chloride needed to address your particular situation, you may experience other symptoms of cancer cell die off. Once again, if you have the luxury of starting slow and progressing slowly than this will lessen any of the potential side effects.

An acidic environment within the cell, as oxygen supplies become depleted, will force the cell to revert to the fermentation of glucose to maintain its energy needs. This metabolic process produces lactic acid which is responsible for a vast majority of the pain associated with cancer. This lactic acid, obviously, increases the acidity of the cell.

Cesium chloride is able to raise the pH level of the cancer cell somewhere between 8.0 and 9.0. The cancer cell soon dies off and is absorbed into the bodily fluids where it will eventually be eliminated.

As Cesium chloride raises the pH of the cell, it consequently shuts down the fermentation process and the buildup of lactic acid. Many patients report a drastic drop or complete relief from the pain associated with these acid deposits and build-up. Some have reported total relief of pain in as little as 1 to 3 days.

The use of cesium chloride and the resulting increase in pH can cause a rapid decline in tumor mass. The material composition of the tumor mass is secreted as uric acid into the urine. It is important to drink adequate amounts of water to assist the kidney's in eliminating these excess acids from the body. Also, the presence of cesium chloride salts in the bodily fluids will generally neutralize a great majority of these acids and render them non-toxic.

Anyone interested in cesium chloride therapy should check into "Essense of Life" online. This company has been helping cancer patients for a long time and have a great ionic product they distribute. They also have a great reputation and very well informed customer support staff. Larry is the man you would want to speak to.

Be careful of any research you read that may be misrepresenting the efficacy of cesium chloride. If you read a report that overly emphasizes the fact that cesium chloride does not kill cancer cells, it is actually somewhat correct. Cesium chloride actually creates the optimal environment for your immune system to kill the cancer cells. It does this by raising the pH of the cell. This blocks or cuts off the fermentation process by raising the oxygen level of the cell and allowing the immune system to finish the job.

There is some debate and differing opinions about the percentage of cancer cells that are destroyed by the use of cesium chloride and the percentage of cells that actually revert from a cancerous cell back into a normal, healthy cell.

Case studies and research determined that a normal cell will typically not take up or ingest the Cesium chloride. Also, for those who are unable to utilize or are restricted in some way from taking the cesium chloride orally, it can be used transdermally (applied to the skin) with the addition of DMSO (dimethyl sulfoxide).

It should be cautioned that DMSO is very efficient and effective but, unfortunately, produces a strong offensive body odor that could become an issue, especially if the patient is continuing to function at work.

Don't you think it a bit odd how populations around the world that have not been subjected to adulterated foods grown in mineral depleted soils are robust and healthy. Cancer is an anomaly for these people. These tribes of people obtain their food from volcanic soils rich in mineral concentrations of potassium, rubidium, cesium and all the other essential minerals.

Could it be that our whole health, sickness issue is tied to a lack of essential minerals and essential vitamins in their perfect, whole, unadulterated, unenhanced, synergistic configuration? Could it be so pathetically simple? Science is continually and exceedingly perplexed in its pursuit of that elusive yet undeniably magical cure.

The water supply of one of the healthiest groups of people worldwide, the Hunza's of Northern Pakistan, has been analyzed and found to be very rich in the mineral cesium. They are mostly vegetarians and consume large quantities of fruit along with an abundant supply of apricots. They also consume the kernel which is rich in vitamin B17 (Laetrile). Hmmmm.

The cost of cesium chloride therapy varies depending on what other additional supplements are deemed necessary and complimentary to your particular situation. The cost for a 1 month supply as of this writing is $175.00. That includes the ionic cesium chloride and ionic potassium supplement.

There are numerous case studies affirming the efficacy of Cesium chloride and its miraculous turnarounds. Many late stage and terminal cancers have been reversed. Even the patients that were given up by conventional medicine and deemed a lost cause.

Unfortunately many still die. It would seem that far too many people decide on an alternative cancer treatment only after conventional medicine has written them off and already, severely poisoned and damaged their systems and or organs, some irrevocably.

When you research the statistics on the efficacy of alternative treatments and how many patients were cured or recovered, you have to take into consideration how many of them came to that alternative treatment via the conventional train of death. It takes the numbers and confidence levels down considerably.

Sad that so many only find their nerve when faced with no other options, a dead end in the hope for recovery. Very sad that for many it is already too late. The nail has been set. It doesn't have to be like this. Why aren't we informed of the successes in alternative therapies. I guess we both know the answer to that. Some of us will keep fighting, others will sadly lay bare their souls and simply fade away. E Pluribus Unum, Caveat Emptor!

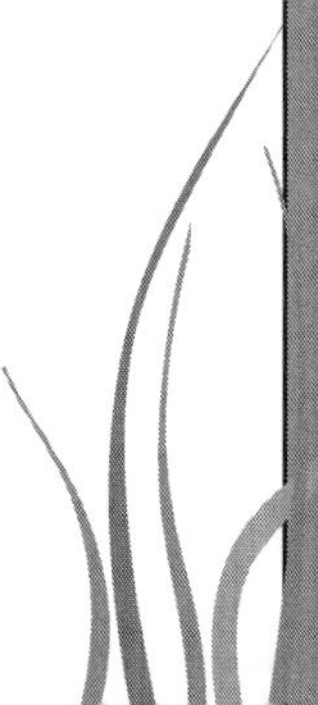

Chapter 16

Protocel/Cancell

Protocel is a non-herbal formula that targets anaerobic cells in the body while leaving normal, healthy cells safe and unaffected. Cancer cells are termed anaerobic because they derive their energy from the fermentation of glucose or sugar, whereas healthy cells derive their energy from oxygen.

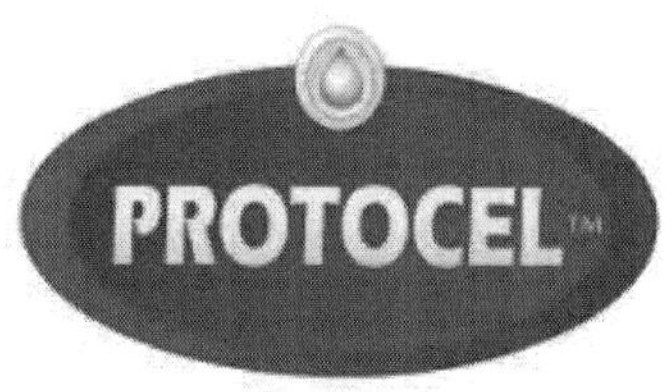

Protocel interferes with the respiration between cancer cells so they cannot receive the energy they need for survival. Since it does not interfere with the respiration or uptake of oxygen, healthy cells are unharmed. This is in huge contrast to chemotherapy where so much internal damage is unfortunately done.

Protocel can usually be purchased at health food stores or you may have to go online. It is sometimes sold as a powerful cell cleanser because of its ability to rid the body of destructive anaerobic cells. These cells are responsible for many chronic diseases.

Protocel is relatively inexpensive and has been used to treat high blood pressure, chronic fatigue, arthritis, multiple sclerosis, fibromyalgia, diabetes and other viral and degenerative diseases.

Since it is such a powerful cell cleanser this rejuvenation and re-birth of healthy cells will have a very profound impact on any bothersome affliction. Again we see the beauty of natural treatments addressing the environment in which the pathogens live and replicate.

The formula was developed by a Pennsylvania chemist. He came from a family of hard working, grit of the Earth, coal miners. He was a very spiritual man and prayed that one day he would somehow be able to help mankind, leaving his mark of benevolence on humanity or even the possibility of finding a cure for cancer. It was in his later years of high school that he began having a recurring dream of a particular chemical formula.

By fate he came across an article in a book that laid out the basis of the formula in his dream. It was an article on known carcinogens and he just happened to open this large book to the exact page. It was a surprising twist of luck or was it fate?

It was during a demonstration in college that a random combining of fluids took place along with a very curious reaction that dumbfounded the other professors in the room also.

Soon after this event, Mr. Sheridan was given a long term project that would invariably change his future, and lead him in a very specific direction. As in his earlier dreams, Sheridan had another dream that unveiled the hypothesis of his studies and the potential factors for his formula.

Sheridan worked on his formula from 1930 -1990. After many many years of trial and error his success rates treating mice continued to grow evermore successful and optimistic. By 1983 he had achieved an 80% cure rate on the rodent cancers used for his research.

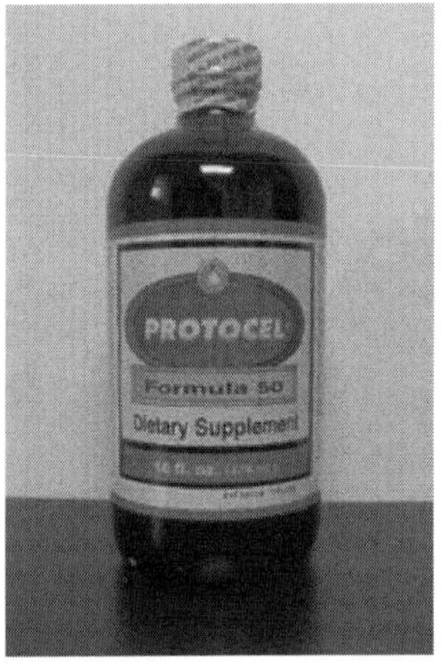

He originally named the formula, Entelev, which stems from the Greek word, Entelechy. It translated to "that part of man known only to God."

Anaerobic cells are not always cancer cells although, any cells in the body that are anaerobic are abnormal, unhealthy, and tend to be associated with a variety of different maladies and afflictions.

The easiest description of how Protocel works is that it effects every cell in the body by biochemically lowering the voltage between cells. That lowered voltage interferes with the production of ATP (adenosine triphosphate), and or your energy source.

Cancer cells already operate at a lower, less efficient energy level than normal cells because they obtain their energy from the fermentation of glucose, instead of the respiration or intake of oxygen.

The 10-15% reduction in voltage created by the Protocel lowers the voltage in the cells just enough, that the cancer or any other anaerobic cell cannot survive and or maintain function. These anaerobic cells break down or "lyse" into a harmless protein. To put it more simply, they just fall apart.

Fortunately, healthy, normal cells are unaffected by this 10-15% reduction in voltage. Healthy aerobic or oxygenated cells operate at such a high level of energy or voltage, a slight drop of this voltage leaves the healthy cell unaffected, whereas, an anaerobic cell is already operating at a low level of energy, and the 10-15% drop in voltage causes the cell to self destruct. It breaks down into a harmless, digestible protein.

The process of this transformation and destruction is called "lysing." When complete, the body will use one of the various routes of elimination to dispose of it. A patient will often see a mucous type material in their feces and urine or, they may even cough up a whitish, mucous like substance.

The good news is that so far, because Protocel targets the respiratory system of anaerobic cancer cells, the cancer cells are unable to mutate or resist its system of destruction.

Chemotherapy drugs on the other hand are often ineffective and the cancer cells are able to mutate and resist it. That is part of the reason why multiple chemotherapy drugs are sometimes administered together or have to be rotated periodically.

As with many forms of alternative cancer therapies, the case histories that are documented, are extremely promising. There is a story of a woman that was diagnosed with a rare form of a nervous system cancer called Glioblastoma Multiforme, stage 4. These types of cancers are typically always fatal.

According to surgeons, the source of her pain was a tumor located on her spinal cord in her thoracic area. The surgery was only partially successful. The tumor was malignant and surgeons were unable to fully res-sect the tumor from her spine.

The patient was told she would now have free floating cancer cells in her spinal fluid and that they would eventually travel to her brain and initiate tumors there also.

Doctor's suggested a very aggressive bone marrow chemotherapy and massive radiation. Either way, the treatments would cause great damage to her body and would only, possibly, extend her life 3-6 months. Her future sadly seemed hopeless.

She and her husband were bombarded with suggestions of various alternative treatments. Fortunately, one of these treatments was Protocel. At the time it was still known as Cancell. Needless to say she was very skeptical, thinking that surely if something as effective as the reports she had been reading were accurate, thousands of people would certainly know about it.

Her husband had Faith and an intuition that the Cancell would work so they decided against conventional treatments, and started on the Cancell. After nearly 3 weeks on the Cancell, she was admitted back into the hospital for some blood abnormalities. They continued administering the Cancell around the clock.

After 3 ½ months of administering the Cancell, they performed new scans of her brain and her spinal column. The results came back 100% negative for any signs of cancer. She continued the Cancell for 2 ½ years to be sure the cancer would not return. As of this writing it has been nearly 20 years since her diagnosis and she remains, to this day, cancer free.

This is just one of several case studies and recoveries attributed to Cancell and or Protocel. It is yet another alternative cancer treatment that has been suppressed by the medical establishment.

Because it posed a threat to the large chemotherapy industry, it was never approved by the FDA. Anything not approved by the FDA will generally fall off into obscurity. Sadly, the majority of doctors will not have any information on its use and or its effectiveness.

In 1953, Jim Sheridan had such success with his Cancell/Protocel formula on laboratory mice that the director of the Detroit Institute of Cancer Research decided it was time to try the formula in a clinical trial.

Sheridan received funding for the trial and was ready to begin when the Detroit director informed the American Cancer Society of the upcoming clinical program.

The American Cancer Society immediately put a stop to the program saying that Sheridan had no proof that he owned the idea. It was a bizarre turn of events and soon after, Jim Sheridan was suspiciously fired from the Detroit Institute of Cancer Research. He later found out that his research, and the results of that research while at the institute, had been destroyed or burned.

He later worked for the bio sciences division of the Battelle Institute. They were a research center where the latest chemotherapy drugs were being tested for the National Cancer Institute.

The chemotherapy tests were conducted in 5 day studies. A Dr. Davidson asked if Sheridan's formula could be tested over a 28 day period as his formula was not a poison. Lessening the respiration between cells took a bit longer to work.

This request was denied by the National Cancer Institute. They refused to allow anything beyond the 5 day trial limit. Sometime in the late 1970's he was able to get the National Cancer Institute to administer his formula to animals.

There were very specific requirements necessary for its proper administration, which Sheridan sent to them personally. For some reason, which was never resolved, the specific requirements were never followed and the National Cancer Institute reported the ineffectiveness of the formula.

Over and over Sheridan tried in any way possible to spread the news of his remarkable discovery only to be denied. The FDA, the National Cancer Institute and the other powers that control the massive chemo industry made sure Cancell/Protocel never reached public awareness.

Certain media outlets that could have brought this formula to the public attention, were threatened with having their licenses revoked if they reported any positive benefits, or other information on Sheridans Cancell/Protocel formula.

Fortunately, an independent businessman, after hearing of the remarkable results with Cancell/Protocel, decided to make it available at no cost to cancer patients that were in need. Legally, there was nothing the Cancer thugs could do being that they were not actually selling Cancell/Protocel but, giving it away.

The effectiveness of the formula was and is without a doubt quite remarkable. The fact that this research and the miraculous recoveries that have been suppressed, is equally and unbelievably amazing. It stifles the imagination. It has more than proven to be completely safe and non-toxic even when taken indefinitely.

Sadly, the toxic, conventional power treatments won the day, even though these conventional treatments typically have to be spaced out because of the extensive damage to the body. Does the chemo or the cancer kill the patient? You might be surprised. Nevertheless, cancer usually grows back in between treatments and it typically grows back fairly quickly. Mostly because the immune system has been obliterated by these life destroying, conventional protocols from hell.

In the end game of the Cancer elite, Sheridan received an FDA court injunction to stop all distribution of Cancell/Protocel completely. They didn't care if he gave it away or not, and the people were once again denied their freedom to choose.

They denied Protocel based on toxicity tests that Sheridan was never able to acquire. The cat and mouse game was way too clever and way too powerful. The kings of cancer would make sure those toxicity tests were never brought to conclusion. That way they could keep it out of sight and out of the hands of the public at large.

There are 2 different formula's of Protocel. Formula 23 and formula 50. They differ very slightly. They are made with the same ingredients but the amount taken is somewhat different. Formula 50 is considered to be a little faster acting and initiates the lysing or dying off effect a bit quicker.

Which one you decide to use would be based on your type of cancer and the urgency of your particular situation. You would also have to keep in mind that the lysing effect can create some edema or swelling. So, if the area your addressing is a confined space such as the brain, it is highly recommended to start slower and try and control any potential swelling that may occur. Having a well educated practitioner is very important especially when dealing with cancers where too much inflammation could be dangerous and even fatal.

It is generally advised to start slowly anyway and stick to a specific timetable and amount for administering the Protocel. It is typically recommended to take 1/8 to 1/4 teaspoon 4 -5 times a day at evenly spaced intervals.

It is best taken on an empty stomach, typically, 30-40 minutes before eating. For any questions on specifics there is a Protocel user support forum that should be able to answer any detailed questions you may have.

It needs to be noted that since Protocel decreases the production of ATP and effects the energy of the cell, herbs and or other supplements that tend to raise (ATP) the energy levels of the cell can interfere with the effectiveness of Protocel.

You can obtain a good amount of added information from the Protocel forum on the supplements to avoid if you decide on this protocol for treatment. It is typically not a problem using Protocel while on a cancer or other disease fighting, alkaline diet. The normal daily allowance of nutrients you receive through the foods you consume should be fine but, certain added supplements need to be avoided while on Protocel.

A few of the herbs and or supplements you should avoid are: Vitamin C, Vitamin E, Ozone Therapy, Essiac Tea, CoQ10 and Selenium. The amounts of these particular vitamins you receive in the food you eat are typically fine, just don't add any extra supplementation.

The use or combining of Ozone therapy along with Protocel should also be avoided. Ozone chemically interacts with the formula and causes toxic by products or aldehydes that can harm the body. Drinking purified bottled water should be fine as the ozone typically used to purify the water has usually dissipated by the time it reaches you.

Other supplements that should be avoided are: Ginseng, L-Cysteine, Glutamine, Glutathione, Taurine, Poly-MVA, Homeopathic medicine, Acetyl-Cysteine, Creatine, Sea Silver, Alpha lipoic acid, L-Carnitine, IP6, Acetyl L-Carnitine and The Rife Machine Protocol.

This is a partial list of supplements that should be Ok while using Protocel: Ellagic acid, Laetrile, Shark liver oil, Grapeseed extract, Fish oils, Coral calcium, Milk thistle, Calcium, Magnesium, Potassium, Reishi mushrooms, Noni juice, Vitamin D3, Soy isoflavones, Collostrum, Hydrazine Sulfate, DMSO, Multi-B Vitamins and any type of Digestive enzyme.

You should receive more information from the vendor of the Protocel. It should be included with your purchase of the product.

The results and recoveries using Protocel are impressive. If you decide that this is the alternative treatment that best suits your particular situation then you need to heed the guidelines. Unless you find documented evidence otherwise, it is best advised to avoid taking anything other than what you would receive in your prescribed diet.

I know this is a very difficult decision. We all have the tendency and upbringing to not trust alternative therapies. After all, the majority of us have been raised thinking them a sham. We have a natural tendency towards combining multiple therapies just in case the one we have chosen doesn't work or, maybe the one we have chosen will have a better chance of working with extra's added in, it's the team mentality thing we have to overcome.

There are many of the described treatments that can be combined much safer than combining with Protocel because of its interaction with the energy production of the cell. The fact of the matter is that Protocel has proven to be highly effective and healing. It's the courage or fear of putting all your eggs in the Protocel basket and trusting that decision.

Apparently Protocel does not interfere with most prescription medications and it typically does not interfere with their effectiveness. Thing is, if you commit to using Protocel, other health conditions are also greatly improved. The dosage and or your need for prescribed, conventional medications is usually drastically reduced or sometimes removed altogether.

Many patients that start on Protocel, stay on the program for up to 2 years after the all clear for cancer has been confirmed. The reports of people that were not successful with Protocel were usually patients that were already so damaged internally from the chemo, radiation or surgery, that their bodies could not produce and sustain a recovery.

Studies have shown that Protocel does not interfere with short term or minimally dosed radiation. It all depends on how much damage has been done to the bodies ability to function, and the state of your vital organs. Some have even benefited from Protocel and low dose radiation, being that they both work on lowering the voltage within the cell.

There is still a lot of controversy on the effectiveness of using Protocel along with chemotherapy. Some types seem to benefit while others do not. That would be a good question to post in the Protocel forum to see what others have experienced.

Protocel may also be administered to pets. There are many stories of people with sick and cancerous dogs, cats and horses that have been completely cured, even in its most advanced stages. Of course the dosage would have to be adjusted accordingly.

The benefit of Protocel is that it will not harm your pets either. Many veterinarians across the U.S. use Protocel as a part of their treatment strategies regularly.

Chapter 17

The Kelmun Protocol

All treatments for cancer need to start with an alkaline diet as the basis for any and all foods you consume. It is proven that a high alkaline diet slows down and even stops the progression of cancer. Remember that a high alkaline diet is an oxygen rich diet. I know you've heard it all before, and that I'm repeating myself, and you'll probably hear it all again but this is so incredibly important.

The Kelmun protocol consists of a combination of aluminum free baking soda and a raw, organic, grade B maple syrup.

It has been used with surprising success. Many people cannot afford the costs and the enormous financial burden needed to sustain some of the natural treatments for any length of time. I should know that best. I lost my house and my business trying to sustain and maintain, beyond my means, alternative therapies.

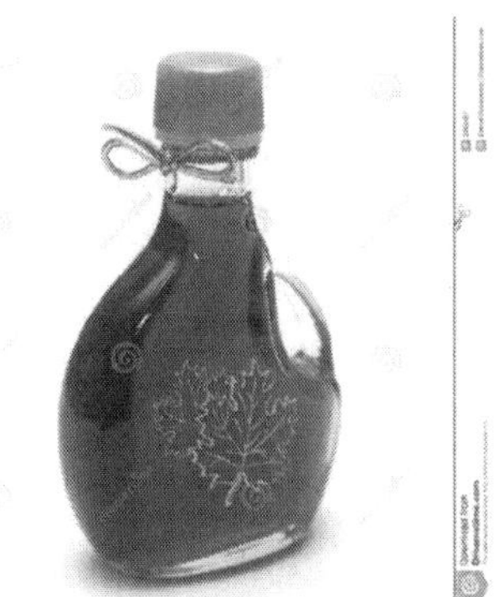

The darker the maple syrup the better. Try and find organic grade B which is normally darker. If that is not available, buy the darkest organic grade A you can find.

The baking soda is very alkaline and is used to raise the pH of the cell thereby, indirectly enabling and initiating the death of the cancer cell. The maple syrup is used as a carrier for the baking soda since cancer cells consume 15 times more glucose (sugar) than normal cells it is the perfect combination. It's kind of like using a piece of candy to coax the cancer to its demise.

Pretty simple concept and strategy. Attach and ingest a substance that cancer hates along with something the cancers cells cannot live without, sugar, and the cancer cell will readily and willingly sap it up.

This is based on other treatments which use a highly alkaline substance to kill the microbes inside of a cancer cell. Baking Soda, Calcium and Cesium Chloride are a few of the alkaline substances used today.

The protocol calls for 1 level teaspoon of aluminum free baking soda and 3 teaspoons of 100% pure, preferably grade B, maple syrup. Be sure to stay away from aluminum pots and pans. Use glass, stainless steel or copper. Never ever use aluminum, if you do have aluminum pots or pans that you use for any cooking, throw them out and be rid of them.

Put the mixture into a pot and heat on low for about 7 minutes or whatever it takes to almost burn the mixture, then, reduce the heat. You want to heat it just enough for the mixtures to blend well. Be sure to stay away from any refined sugar or refined flour products so the cancer cells take up as much of the baking soda/ maple syrup combination as possible.

Take 1 teaspoon of the mixture at a time, in fact it is best to start with 1 teaspoon a day for a couple of days then, try taking 2 teaspoons. Space them out 1 at a time and wait 2-4 hours before taking a second teaspoon. Do not take more than 3 teaspoons daily.

This is a very simple and obviously basic, inexpensive remedy people and other healthcare professionals have used many times with surprising results, although this information has been very quietly acknowledged.

The Kelmun Protocol is the story of a man who was treating cancer patients that had nowhere else to go. They did not have the funding or monies for some of the other more expensive alternative therapies.

His successes continued to get attention, unfortunately, they also got the attention of the local media. The media posted his story and soon thereafter he was threatened with arrest if he continued to dispense this remedy or any information regarding the formula.

This too, along with most other successful alternative therapies was blasted as quackery, and the public was advised by those in authority and power to ignore this bogus, unsubstantiated, ridiculous claim.

It seems to have worked. I do not know of anyone who has ever heard of this poor man's protocol for treating cancer, let alone, ever used it. There are quite a few testimonials that seem quite valid along with validation from a number of doctors before the intended threats were put into play.

I know, anyone can write a bogus testimonial on any subject on the planet, just as sure as the ones in authority can write the same bogus testimonials, and discredit any alternative that takes money away from their thriving, mainstream, medical establishment.

Eventually you have to end up trusting someone or something otherwise we cannot evolve. There are surely more true to the Divine, suffering patriots than there are sociopathic, greedy, self serving and bigoted egomaniacs.

This is a very inexpensive protocol. A lot of patients combine this therapy along with a couple of the other inexpensive therapies.

There is or was a doctor, I believe an Italian physician, that started administering baking soda directly into cancer sites in the body by means of injection. He had incredible success and reversals of cancer but, when he brought this information and potential cure before the conventional medical authorities in Italy, he was more or less labeled a quack and a lunatic, and I believe they revoked his medical license.

Chapter 18

Hydrogen Peroxide Therapy

The majority of you have never heard of hydrogen peroxide as a cancer therapy. Most only know it as an effective protocol for cleaning out the potential for infection in cuts and scrapes. There is a reason you have never heard of its other applications. There is way too much bad information out there making it difficult to sort through the chaff from the wheat.

Hydrogen Peroxide has been used for well over 100 years to treat a large number of various illnesses. Since it is based on the premise of adding oxygen to the body and bloodstream, its mechanism of action is well documented and understood.

Not only is the abundance of oxygen critical and mandatory for our health, it is a systemic, whole body necessity. It is not a therapy that targets a specific body part or organ. It works on the premise of allowing the body to do the work by giving it the most crucial element necessary for our survival, oxygen.

H_2O_2

Most have never heard of food grade hydrogen peroxide. The basic hydrogen peroxide sold at your local retailer should never be ingested internally. It has far too many added chemicals and stabilizers. It must be food grade, 35% hydrogen peroxide diluted down to a 3% solution. Full strength 35% hydrogen peroxide can burn your skin.

The hardest thing about inexpensive and simple remedies for cancer is just that, it is so simple it sounds ridiculous. Most people will more or less tune you out once you mention hydrogen peroxide and cancer in the same sentence. It is so infuriating when we have been so cleverly conditioned to dismiss anything beyond or out of mainstream conceivability.

It also doesn't cost enough. I mean, how could anything so ridiculously inexpensive conquer something so malevolent as cancer. That's our logic, right? It is so far from being even remotely believable we quickly forget and erase the very thought of it from our minds. If someone told you that you could treat your cancer or other illness for about $1.50 a day would you even pay attention. I probably wouldn't either.

We need to grasp the larger picture. We need to look beyond and understand the mechanism of action, added oxygen. We need to see it for what it really is. It is another way of adding oxygen to our ever decreasing and polluted supply. Such an enormously simple concept don't you think?

This is a therapy for those that are not financially able to support other alternative treatments. It can result in penny's a day to administer instead of thousands. Just because it is cheap does nothing to erase or decrease its chances for success.

The beauty of this simplistic approach is that it relies on the innate sense and brilliance of our own body. What I'm trying to say is that it not only has the potential to treat, reverse and or heal cancer but, any other crux that might be dragging down your quality of life.

As I have stated before, the biggest reason you have never heard of this therapy is because you cannot patent oxygen, therefore, there is no financial incentive to spread the word. In fact, spreading the word would kill a lot of voluminous, overflowing, superabundant bank accounts. It would be a huge and devastating blow to our medically endowed economy.

So, for these players, it really comes down to choosing between your family member potentially dying or keeping the new Lexus and spa membership. The majority of those in the financial loop of deception will discreetly and very selectively contact an alternative practitioner for alternative treatments rather than subject their loved one to the poisons many associate with conventional therapies.

The use of hydrogen peroxide as a vehicle to reclaimed health has been, through numerous successful applications, reported as being completely safe. The only caution is for anyone that has undergone an organ transplant. Hydrogen Peroxide stimulates the immune system with extra oxygen which, in turn, attacks anything deemed foreign within the body. It's use could cause the organ to be rejected so it is not recommended under these circumstances.

The diseases and conditions associated with oxygen deficiency and deprivation are numerous beyond measure. The majority of our so wonderfully labeled afflictions are linked, in one way or another, to some form of oxygen starvation. The majority of diseases are caused, created and sustained by bacteria, viruses, fungi, parasites and other pathogens. It is scientifically proven that nearly all can be eradicated by the very presence and abundance of oxygen.

From AIDS to acne, allergies, arthritis, headaches, heart disease, Epstein-barr, type II diabetes, hepatitis, herpes, lupus, MS, Parkinson's, digestive disorders, ulcers, colitis, cirrhosis of the liver, periodontal disease, Alzheimers, angina and cancer to name just a few. Of course they have all been labeled as independent, isolated conditions with a very conveniently assigned menu of prescribed pharmaceuticals.

The big question is, are these prescribed pharmaceutical medications doing anything to correct your condition or are they simply making them more comfortable and convenient to live with? What do you have to lose? Your affliction???

With hydrogen peroxide therapy there are very limited side effects unless you abuse the suggested dosages and amounts. Even then, if you do experience any side effects, they will be from your body destroying errant pathogens too quickly and dumping them back into your bloodstream.

That's what happens when you detox faster than your body can effectively eliminate the toxins. You still win, you just experience some uncomfortable symptoms for a little while. So, you back off a little and bask in the knowledge that your body is actually under construction and repair.

Hydrogen peroxide has even been used successfully to treat alcoholism. Alcohol impairs the cellular uptake of oxygen creating a deficiency within the cell. By taking hydrogen peroxide orally it helps to saturate the body with increased oxygen and repair cellular respiration. This increased oxygen supply and restored cellular respiration of oxygen actually decreases the cravings for alcohol. Continued use of hydrogen peroxide eventually transforms and removes the body's desire and addiction to the substance altogether.

Its applications are growing more ambitious everyday by those courageous enough to offer it as an option. Because of its ability to saturate the body with increased oxygen, many brain and nerve related illnesses are also being treated and reversed with impressive success.

Dentists are also using hydrogen peroxide to treat a wide variety of periodontal issue's including, gum disease, gingivitis, cavity prevention, bacterial infections and mouth sores.

The biggest problem will be finding a medical practitioner willing to give up that big paycheck that comes along with conventional applications, and offering up the option that rewards him little monetarily. You will have to find the practitioner who signed on for humanity. They survive by making large deposits in a bank account of the heart.

The physicians and researchers in the know and those who have benefited from its application agree that hydrogen peroxide is a viable medical procedure that may be the greatest healing phenomena of all time, manna from heaven.

There are several different grades of hydrogen peroxide. If you plan on administering it at home, which most people do, you need to purchase 35% food grade hydrogen peroxide. This is the only type you can safely ingest internally. This 35% grade will need to be diluted to a 3% solution before taking it internally. This is extremely important!

Most company's that supply 35% food grade hydrogen peroxide will include a dropper bottle and a pair of surgical type gloves. You need to wear the gloves when filling the dropper bottle as 35% food grade peroxide will burn your skin. It's the hydrogen part of the equation. Rinse immediately with water if this occurs.

There are various ways to administer it. If you decide to make a nasal or mouth spray it will still, obviously, need to be diluted to a 3% solution. Use only distilled water for this process.

It is highly advised to start slowly and work up to a higher dose. Once you fill your dropper bottle with the 35% grade hydrogen peroxide you need to mark the bottle and make sure anyone and everyone knows it can be dangerous and even fatal at that concentration and must be diluted before being used.

The beginning dose is 3 drops of the 35% grade diluted into 6-8 ounces of distilled water 3 times a day. It should be taken on an empty stomach, 1 hour before a meal or 2-3 hours after a meal. If it causes any discomfort or nausea cut back on your dosage or re-distribute the same amount of drops in 5 or 6 glasses of water during the day.

It is very important to consume adequate amounts of water while using this protocol. The water will benefit the bodies ability to eliminate dying and dead cellular debris. The peroxide can react with the bacteria in your gut so that is why it is best to administer it on an empty stomach.

It can have an odd, unappetizing flavor especially as you increase the amount of drops daily. You can either wash it down with some other liquid, more water or add some juice or other flavor to the distilled water to make it more palatable.

The directions are to increase the amount of drops by 1 for each glass, 3 times a day. In other words start at 3 drops in 6-8 oz. of distilled water 3 times a day on the first day, moving up to 4 drops in 6-8 oz. of distilled water 3 times a day on the second day, progressing to 5 drops in 6-8 oz. of distilled water 3 times a day on the third day and so on.

Keep increasing 1 drop in each glass 3 times a day, each day, until you reach 25 drops in 6-8 oz of distilled water 3 times a day. Depending on the severity of your illness you can choose to move slower. Determine whether or not your body is effectively eliminating the oxidized, dead cellular debris. You will be able to tell by how you are feeling. You need to make sure your bowels are also working efficiently, this is extremely important.

When I did it, I went extremely slow. I wasn't fighting any major affliction so I had the luxury of going super slow. I did 3 drops in 8 ounces of distilled water once a day for 3-4 days. I then increased to 4 drops in 8 ounces of distilled water once a day for 3-4 days. I think this is a good way to go to avoid uncomfortable side effects as much as possible. Again it will all depend on what affliction you are fighting and how much time you have available. I also made sure to drink extra water. Remember half your weight in ounces should be your goal for daily water consumption.

Once you reach the goal of 25 drops in 6-8 oz of distilled water 3 times a day, do the same as you did on the way up but in reverse. Decrease 1 drop in each glass of water 3 times a day, each day, until you reach the starting point of 3 drops in 6-8 oz of distilled water 3 times a day. This is considered a maintenance dose and should be continued indefinitely depending on your affliction.

Anyone battling a very severe medical condition should stay on the 25 drops, 3 times a day for up to 3 weeks and then, decrease down by 1 less drop a day in each glass until you reach the recommended maintenance dose.

Warning: After deciding to use hydrogen peroxide as a treatment for your affliction you need to pay very close attention to your symptoms and how you feel. The extra oxygen in your body is going to start the healing and cleansing process of oxidation. Depending on how toxic you are, the symptoms and or side effects can be quite uncomfortable. Many people stop the therapy simply because at times they may feel worse. This is usually a sign that the process is working.

This is what happens when your body starts breaking down and eliminating toxic debris. Many people will start with just the 3 drops of 35% hydrogen peroxide in 6-8 oz of distilled water once a day for 3 days, then, slowly increase to 3 drops, 2 times a day and so on. You do not want to go too fast. If you have the luxury of doing it in baby steps then it is usually recommended to do so. It is your choice, monitor closely how you feel. Detoxing can come with flu like symptoms, fever, nausea, aches and pains and so on, it's part of the package.

Also, remember you need to complete the program once you start. Once the oxygen starts to do its work, it is vitally important for it to be able to finish that work. Many people have quit half way through the protocol only to have more issue's than they had before.

Dead, dying and destroyed cellular waste getting stirred up from the oxygen doing its work will sometimes settle elsewhere within the body. If you quit the program too early, it can cause an issue to manifest elsewhere that wasn't there before.

You need to continue and finish the program the way it was designed. Did you really think it was going to be a cakewalk out of toxicity, out of dis-ease. We have been abusing our bodies for far to long. We have been asking it to function without the proper ingredients. We continually add, on a daily basis, more and more foreign, what the hell am I supposed to do with this, anomalous muck.

This protocol is very effective and has had unbelievable results when administered correctly under the supervision of an educated medical practitioner. Since it is not a mainstream conventional therapy, finding a medical practitioner willing to supervise this process will be difficult. The majority have never even heard of this protocol, it certainly isn't taught in our medical schools.

It is illegal to practice medicine without a license or with anything relating to cancer. The only legal treatment being surgery, radiation or chemotherapy. It would be advised to seek out the opinion of a practitioner trained in the practice of alternative therapies. Even then, most will only be able to offer advice since many are not licensed to prescribe.

Chapter 19

Wheatgrass Therapy

The health benefits of wheatgrass was discovered back in 1925 by a Dr. Charles Schnabel. Other medical doctors and scientists were also involved in the discovery and research of wheatgrass. Ann Wigmore re-discovered these benefits and popularized it back in the 1970's. In fact Ann Wigmore founded the Hippocrates Health Institute which is still going strong with her Living Foods Lifestyle.

Dr. Schnabel was an agricultural chemist and his primary purpose was determining the value and benefits of various animal feeds and which ones had the greatest benefit to livestock production.

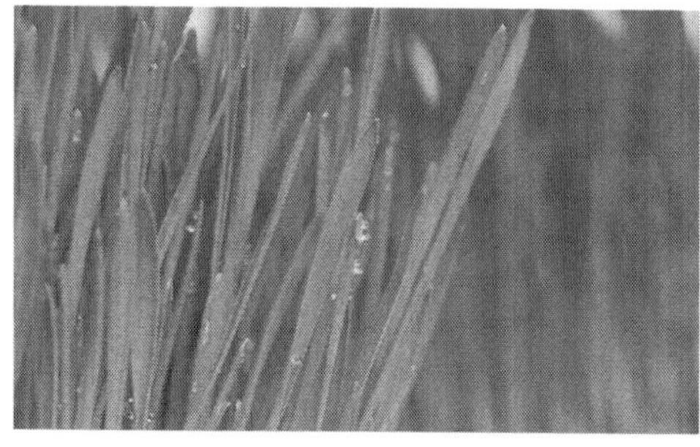

They already knew of the amazing results of livestock that were allowed to graze on wheatgrass in the spring. The livestock raised for beef showed remarkable weight gain. The dairy cows increased in milk production and butter fat increased by more than 30%.

It was in an interview that Dr. Schnabel's son told the story of a day when his father walked out into the wheatgrass field. The wheatgrass was only 8 inches tall and he decided to harvest some of it by hand with a pair of scissors. This wheatgrass had been planted the previous fall in some very fertile, alluvial, glacial soil in northeast Kansas.

He took what he had cut back to the house and dried it. He then mixed a very small amount (6%) into some chicken feed and documented the results. Surprisingly, the hens in the study went from an egg production rate of 30% up to 90%. Hens that had been laying an egg every 3 days started laying an egg almost everyday. This exciting news started a very intense period of research for food scientists.

Dr. Schnabel knew that cereal grasses were a rich source of chlorophyll as they were a much darker green than the other plants and vegetables. The research confirmed that the darker the green the more chlorophyll it contained.

Dr. Schnabel then developed a low temperature drying process that quickly removed the moisture from the fresh wheatgrass. Part of this process involved a rotating drum. The temperature of the wheatgrass after the dehydration process was the same temperature as the surrounding air. This low temperature process was used to preserve all the vital nutrients and enzymes.

With all the human research going on, the animal research also continued. Several reports from Gynecologists found that giving this dehydrated cereal grass to human mothers produced more milk and a richer milk. Researchers also found that by giving only a small percentage of dehydrated cereal grasses (about 6%) to their hogs, cows, horses, sheep and goats, that they produced the same results; more milk, richer milk, much healthier babies and less infant mortality.

This dehydrated cereal grass was made into tablets and somewhere around 1932, "Cerophyl" was born. The science at the time determined that 20 of these cereal grass tablets was equal to the minimum daily requirement of vitamins and minerals. It was, some would say our first multivitamin.

The sales of Cerophyl took off. Pharmacies in the U.S. and in other countries around the world, routinely stocked Cerophyl. Medical doctors began prescribing Cerophyl to their patients from all the various medical reports confirming the positive results when added to the diet. Gynecologists, ophthalmologists, dentists and many other various medical professionals reported similar, positive results.

By 1939, the American Medical association published a report in the Journal of the American Medical Association accepting dehydrated cereal grass as a food. This was published as a result of all the positive and impressive documentation that was pouring in.

In the late 1940's, Cerophyl sales began to decline with the new and improved 1 a day, synthetic multivitamin taking over the spotlight. It was a miracle of modern science. It didn't matter at the time for the unassuming public whether it was all natural or not. That was well before the natural vs. synthetic consciousness was even considered. The public was too mesmerized and focused on the wonders of modern technology and the amazing feat of putting all our recommended daily allowance of vitamins and minerals into 1 little tablet. Oh, those were the days, ugh!

Dr Schnabel and other scientists continued to research the potency of wheatgrass at various stages of growth. At the jointing stage the nutrient concentration dropped off. The jointing stage is when the microscopic grain ovule begins its journey moving up from the roots inside of a developing stalk. So now, the nutritional components are being utilized in the development of the grain and the nutritional power of the grass begins to decline.

Surprisingly, wheatgrass and other cereal grasses have a very similar nutrient composition to other dark green leafy vegetables, but they have it in much greater concentrations.

The scientists found no discernible differences in the nutrient value of the different young grasses (wheat, barley and rye), but each had an escalating nutrient value up until the jointing stage, followed by a rapid decline as the grain developed inside of the stalk. The biggest difference in nutritional density was where the cereal grasses were grown. Nothing compared to the mineral rich, glacial soil found in northeastern Kansas. Back to that mineral depleted soil thing again, yes?

Science remains somewhat mystified as to what nutrients cereal grasses contain that other vegetables and greens do not. In a controlled study back in 1939, animals were fed a diet rich in green vegetables, carrots and spinach. Only one of the 2 groups had a small amount of dehydrated cereal grasses added to their diet. Each time, the results were the same.

The animals that received that small amount of added cereal grasses, grew faster, larger and had greater overall health as shown by their rich coats, eyes and energy levels.

They discovered that a very important hormone found in wheatgrass, abscisic acid, was only present in dehydrated wheatgrass grown throughout the winter in colder weather. They believe that this abscisic acid is what regulates and slows the growth of cereal grasses in winter. They also determined that the abscisic acid was the reason why wheatgrass grown an average of 200 days throughout the winter, was still shorter than wheatgrass grown indoors. Strange that the winter wheatgrass grown for 200 days was still shorter than wheatgrass grown indoors for 10 days.

Sorry for the wheatgrass juice bars. If you want the full effects and the full healing potential of wheatgrass, the dehydrated wheatgrass grown throughout the winter in these mineral rich, volcanic soils, is going to be more potent than the fresh, straight from the flat wheatgrass grown indoors. It all comes down to the additional abscisic acid component.

Scientists speculate that since this abscisic acid slows the growth of the cereal grasses, than this might be the component that is effective in slowing the growth of tumors. Hopeful, but it is still based on theory.

Wheatgrass is an amazing super food. It has a long list of benefits to the body and our health. It helps to cleanse the blood, organs and the gastrointestinal tract of toxic debris. It has been used successfully to treat colitis, constipation, peptic ulcers, indigestion and other issue's affecting the gastrointestinal tract.

Wheatgrass helps to correct an over acidic bloodstream by restoring it to an alkaline state. It increases our red blood cell count and helps to dilate the pathways of the blood thereby decreasing blood pressure.

Wheatgrass also helps to cleanse and clear the lymphatic system. It helps to remove heavy metals, restores vitality to the liver and kidneys, fights cancerous tumors, neutralizes toxins and environmental pollutants and stimulates the thyroid gland.

Wheatgrass is rich in chlorophyll which is very similar to our own hemoglobin. Hemoglobin carries oxygen in the blood. Chlorophyll helps to increase hemoglobin production which in turn increases the amount of oxygen available in the blood which in turn strengthens the immune system and its ability to destroy cancerous microbes.

Wheatgrass is one of the most alkaline foods on the planet. It is rich in a plethora of nutrients and enzymes including several antioxidant vitamins, minerals and amino acids.

It contains the antioxidant enzyme SOD (superoxide dismutase) which converts a very dangerous free radical ROS (reactive oxygen species) into a hydrogen peroxide molecule and an oxygen molecule. It also helps to lessen the effects of radiation. There are over 30 different enzymes in wheatgrass.

One of the most important of these enzymes is cytochrome oxidase. In 1938, a well known cancer researcher and scientist, Paul Gerhardt Seeger, M.D., revealed what he believed to be the true cause of the cancerous degeneration of a cell. He believed that it resulted from the destruction of a specific respiratory enzyme, cytochrome oxidase. The destruction of this enzyme, according to Dr. Seeger interfered with the utilization and respiration of oxygen.

Isn't it amazing how oxygen and our lack of oxygen seems to be the key player in just about every successful therapy? Too bad, it seems that everyday we deplete more and more of the Earth's ability to produce more disease destroying oxygen. That doesn't lessen our need for it, our ever increasing and absolute need for it. We simply must, everyday, find ways to supplement our lives and bodies with oxygen enriching whole supplements, food and water.

Many believe it is the chlorophyll in wheatgrass that is the most effective against cancer. Chlorophyll is what gives green plants their color. Chlorophyll is the molecule that absorbs the suns light and initiates photosynthesis, the conversion of water and CO_2 into energy producing carbohydrates.

From all the research and experiments using cereal grasses, scientists to this day are still mystified as to what nutrients and compound components the cereal grasses contain that other highly beneficial plant based foods do not. The scientists referred to this phenomena as "the unidentified vitamins of cereal grasses," also known as the "grass juice factor."

For now the mystery remains veiled in speculation and theory. All you need to know is that these theories, so far, have been profound in their whole food application for animals as well as for humans. The results prove its power to increase health and defend against disease.

If you decide to use wheatgrass as part of your therapy it is crucial to purchase it from a reputable and well educated source. The wheatgrass commonly purchased in flats and the kind you typically find in a health food stores in liquid shots, does not contain this very important acid. It's still loaded with nutrition but for cancer therapy the addition of abscisic acid should be part of your protocol.

If you remember from earlier in this article, only cereal grasses grown in this type of soil through the cold winter months contains the very important hormone abscisic acid. It is critical, especially if you are treating cancer that you obtain wheatgrass that has been properly cultivated, harvested and definitely connected to the Earth through the winter.

There are a couple of different companies that still grow and dehydrate wheatgrass through the long cold winter in mineral rich soils. You shouldn't have any problem finding a quality product.

Chapter 20

Flaxseed Oil and Cottage Cheese

This is another simplistic yet very logical approach to treating cancer and other afflictions, working from the ground floor up. Too simple I guess for my first wife to get her head around. I couldn't quite figure out her reasons or her thinking.

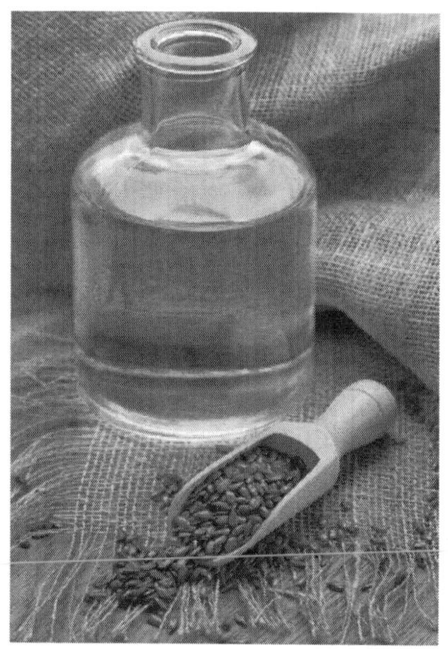

I tried like crazy to try and get her to eat the flax-seed oil and cottage cheese mixture. Unrefined cold processed flax-seed oil is rich in linoleic acid and alpha-linolenic acid, both essential fatty acids crucial to good cellular health.

I don't know at this point if the brain cancer had already altered her thinking processes or if she had just had enough of the fighting and finally relinquished to the idea that she was going to die. It broke my heart when she would not try this creation. I even ate the mixture myself and offered to eat it with her every time.

I pleaded with her, this is your life, it's actually pretty good, what if it really works? It made sense to me. It's always the simple approaches that so many people dismiss as illogical and ludicrous. After all, our current medical system has the cancer enigma clouded in an aura of doom and gloom. We are dumbfounded with the impression that it must be extraordinarily difficult and enormously expensive to overcome.

Something so inane and commonplace treating the most virulent epidemic of modern times? It almost sounds laughable if it wasn't for the science behind the effect. It's also takes a lot more Faith, belief and determination to even consider something so common.

Sadly, many are defeated before they even give themselves a chance. Most everyone eventually dies once they have a confirmed diagnosis, right? Wrong, you die when you decide mentally, in your heart and in your soul that it has you beat.

Other than a Divine intervention from God, too many succumb mentally to the very idea of cancer. Many are dead very close to when their esteemed doctors estimate they will die. They convince their mind that their beloved doctor is some almighty seer that can somehow predict their final days.

That's how the majority of us were raised, with a smug, innate, misplaced confidence that says, hey, my Doc says there's nothing more he can do, so he sent me home to die! Need to get my affairs in order. How many times have you heard that one? Its so hard to break that long standing, ingrained, sealed with a kiss mentality!!!

This is a chapter that will enlighten you on the protocol of treating cancer through an odd yet very effective combination. I know it seems far fetched, it's like saying that eating 2 lemons, 3 purple grapes and a cup of English tea every morning at 8 o'clock and one at 12:30 will remedy insanity or something. Really? Sometimes it is astonishing when something so simple can have such dramatic results.

First of all, omega 3"s and omega 6's are what make up our essential fatty acids. Essential means that the body does not manufacture these crucial fats, and that we need to obtain these essential fats from the foods we eat.

A German biochemist named Johanna Budwig began research in the 1950's on the importance of essential fatty acids. Through her research she documented the importance of these crucial acids and the lack of these essentials in our modern day diet.

Food manufacturers chemically alter the oils found in many products to keep them from going rancid. By chemically altering the oils, the products that contain them are kept safe for long term storage and extended shipping layovers.

Bottom line once again is, the hell with our health, how can we give the consumer what they want and still keep our profits in the black? I'm sure nearly everyone by now has heard of the damaging effects of hydrogenated oils on our health, arteries and blood pressure. Why? What exactly are hydrogenated oils and why are they so harmful? They are very destructive, chemically altered fats. They are definitely not essential and they definitely don't serve a need in our body.

Dr. Budwig studied the blood samples of patients that were seriously ill with cancer and other degenerative diseases, then, compared their blood to the blood of healthy individuals. What she found was a greenish yellow substance in the blood of the seriously ill patients that was not in the blood of the healthy patients. Hmmmm

She attributed these substances to a severe deficiency of unrefined and natural, essential fatty acids in the blood. These EFA's are critical in the oxygenation of our cells and in maintaining a healthy cell wall and membrane. Wouldn't hurt to read that again, the critical part.

All our cells are covered with a protective layer of fats. They also play a role in the functions going on inside of our cells. You can imagine the breakdown of function in cell creation and process when we are deficient in these absolutely critical fatty acids and plentiful in the altered, man-made, foreign, what the hell do I do with these fatty acids.

This creates abnormal cell growth and cell division. Lipid veins inside the cells influence nutrient delivery and are considered the nerves of the cell. They use electrical impulses within the cell to communicate.

Dr. Budwig believed that the lack of the proper essential fatty acids in the cell membrane resulted in abnormal cell division, not excessive cell growth. In the absence of the proper essential fatty acids to complete the process of cell replication and division, one of our most vital and continuous processes goes awry and the initiation sequence of disease begins.

Cell respiration and the binding of oxygen is the key to life and healthy cell function. A healthy cell membrane will be plentiful in unsaturated, unrefined, essential fatty acids. These healthy, unsaturated fatty acids have an abundant supply of unbound electrons looking for something to bind to.

They have a natural affinity for oxygen. In simple, easy to understand terminology, these unbound electrons are lusting for a beautiful and shapely oxygen molecule to mate with. It's just the way it is. So oxygen will always be what they seek out. This binding to the oxygen stimulates respiration and the health of the cell. It is a beautiful thing when you can feed the cell what it is crying out for, what it has to have to perform.

Part of the reason why unrefined, organic, cold pressed virgin flaxseed oil is so beneficial is that it is electron rich. When it is absorbed into the cell it easily and quite prolifically binds to oxygen and proteins.

When the oils are chemically refined and altered like the oils typically found in your local supermarket, the processing destroys this vital electron cloud thus, inhibiting its ability to assimilate and bind oxygen at and in the cell.

Not only does the refining destroy this crucial electron cloud but these inorganic refined fats end up as disease causing deposits all over the body, including; vital organs, the heart muscle and arteries. This is not conducive to good health but I'm sure you were already thinking in that direction. It will slowly but surely, literally, kill you.

These processed, refined fats are not water soluble when bound to proteins and end up impeding circulation and the free flow of blood and lymphatic fluid. Part of the reason your blood pressure is so high.

It is critical to avoid these life destroying, refined fats and hydrogenated or partially hydrogenated oils, also known as trans fatty acids. This is not something that you can dismiss as just being another bad thing, and oh, I better try and cut way back and try to stay away from them. It is your lifeline to living without disease, without cancer, a body at peace, free of disease and free to perform the way it was designed.

I know you have all heard of the good cholesterol, bad cholesterol diets and healthcare markers foretelling your future fate. The problem with these trans fatty acids is that they are very similar to our good cholesterol, and the body mistakenly uses this oxygen depleted trans fatty acid to build cell membranes. This turns off the whole, electrically charged, electrons attracting oxygen system down. Think about it, read that again or just try and remember, shuts it down.

So what happens when the normal cycle and function of unsaturated, unrefined essential fatty acids attracting and binding to oxygen stops functioning? The cell and its environment become more and more anaerobic, which means absence of oxygen or oxygen starved. What happens when you starve something? Sure, it doesn't die right away but it's energy is waning and death is knocking at the door, your door.

This damaged cell membrane also interferes with the transfer of nutrients and the exchange of cellular waste. Man-made fats create the perfect environment for cancer and other pathogens to thrive. Remember that greenish-yellow substance from earlier, that's your man-made fats on drugs.

Dr. Otto Warburg proved this theory by consistently inducing the development of cancer by reducing the levels of oxygen in the tissues approximately 35%. That means that cancer developed 100% of the time.

Essential fatty acids are also required for the production of Prostaglandins. Essential fatty acids are converted into these hormone like substances and these substances play a major role in regulating several different body mechanisms and functions.

They play such a vital role in so many different parts of the body. They help lower risk factors for cardiovascular disease, improve brain function, behavior, intelligence, mood, and they aid in weight reduction by increased energy levels and appetite suppression. They are necessary to help regulate and assist our endocrine system, nervous system development, improve digestion, decrease infection, speed recovery and healing and help to produce beautiful hair, skin, nails and strong bones.

They also help to regulate blood pressure, our immune response, inflammatory issues, kidney function, the flexibility and pliability of our blood vessels and they help in the metabolism of cholesterol. I could go on but I think you get the point, they are essential and actually, to put it more accurately, mandatory to our long term health and our chances for living life without some dreadful disease.

It's really a big thing. You need to keep this in the forefront of your mind at all times. Pay attention to what you are putting in your body. The right fats play a major role in how you feel and the quality of your life experience. It's all a very carefully orchestrated dance.

What effect will what you put into your body cause or create? So many simple things we sadly put out of our consciousness. We so easily surrender to pleasures and succumb to our addictive appetites. So many things we could and should have avoided somewhere along the line.

Nobody else is looking out for your health but you. Of course there are those seemingly soft jabs from your family and friends about your weight or how you look, but other than that, you are responsible for how well you live and how well you die.

Food manufacturers are in the game of making money. They are not at all concerned about the quality of your life experience and how what they create will affect you somewhere down the road, they are in it for the right now, show me the money right now.

It's time we turned the tables around and focused on what will profit us. You can't dance around your bodies requirements and wait for the blade to drop and then, out of panic, make the changes that could have been so easily adopted a long time ago. What if it's too late. The majority of us are overly and quite irresponsibly, proficient procrastinators. We wait, don't we? We'll start tomorrow.

I think it is inspiring that there are finally a few pioneers of truth that are finally bringing this travesty of fraud into the public spotlight. The massive cover up of how harmful these adulterated foods really are. These frauds the food manufacturers have so cleverly marketed to the passive and unassuming public are finally being exposed. My hat is off to those few who have so courageously enlightened the masses even with the threat of great bodily harm for their public exposure and jaw dropping revelations.

Now that you know a little bit more about Essential Fatty Acids and how extremely important they are to our state of health, you will better understand why and how this simple remedy has been so effective for so many people.

I am not suggesting or advising that you use this as a stand alone remedy for cancer, although, many have had great successes and complete recoveries using this protocol. It certainly will change you immensely from the inside out. Just the basics of how it works should stimulate some curiosity now that you understand how vitally important and crucial to life these essential fats are.

I know you are probably wondering where the cottage cheese comes into the picture. Sounds a bit silly but, Dr. Budwig discovered that the quickest way to effectively re-populate our bodies and cells with the proper essential fatty acids was with the addition of a sulfur based protein.

Dr. Budwig discovered that the bodies ability to utilize these fatty acids was greatly enhanced when they were combined and bonded to a sulfur based protein.

Flaxseed oil is one of the richest sources of essential fatty acids. Dr. Budwig then searched for the richest source of food that was

sulfur based, and that would effectively attach to the flaxseed oil. The goal was the quickest and most efficient delivery system into our tissues and cells.

Since her first choice, Quark, was typically only available in Germany at the time, she decided on cottage cheese since it is readily available worldwide. Once the flaxseed oil was whipped and bound to the sulfur based protein in cottage cheese, it became water soluble and easily bio-available to the body.

She also recommended a diet rich in the B vitamins, vitamin C and a well balanced mineral supplement. These would benefit the effectiveness of the blend. Again, stressing the importance of a well balanced, alkaline diet.

Researchers reported that the use of flaxseed oil alone without the addition of a sulfur based protein, and complimentary co-factor supplementation could even cause some harm. Part of the reason for a balance of additional, whole food supplementation.

I am a firm and die hard believer in whole food supplements. From many years of documented research, taking stand alone, isolated minerals and vitamins can be equally dangerous to your health. You need to supplement with whole foods and supplements balanced the way our Creator designed them, in the proper proportions and percentages.

When you take a legitimate, organic, whole food supplement, carefully and systematically created so as not to destroy vital enzymes and other precious micro-nutrients, you can forget about the "recommended daily allowance." God doesn't make mistakes, take your supplements the way God designed them! All together now.

We lost the balance when man decided he could re-invent the wheel. When man decided what our mineral and vitamin ratio's should be. I trust that God put those ratio's together perfectly when He packaged our original food supply. But, then again, it's that multi-billion dollar vitamin supplement industry that keeps the lies and our eyes diverted elsewhere. Extremely clever and massively effective marketing.

I do believe in some cases and in some extremes, supplements are necessary, but any time you can take your RDA's, pre-packaged in food or in a wholly and completely balanced supplement, the better.

Dr. Budwig found that the greenish yellow substance found in patients blood that were sick slowly disappeared after about 3 months of staying true to her prescribed protocol of flaxseed oil and cottage cheese. It was a way of slowly but surely re-building the body dynamic through the simple but extraordinarily basic, bottom of the barrel, human cell. Huge, life saving gifts sometimes do come in microscopic packages, it's not always what's behind door number 2.

This simple yet very effective modality can transform and begin the healing process from a wide range of degenerative conditions including cancer. If you remember what we just talked about, there is extensive research by top scientists that positively prove cancer and other microbes of death and destruction absolutely despise oxygen, it is their supreme nemesis.

So the simple action of feeding your body the essential fatty acids, unrefined, organic, the way nature created them with simplicity of design, works like magic. These oils are electron rich and draw oxygen to themselves. They are the building blocks of a healthy, disease free, oxygen rich, pathogen destroying super cell.

Oxygen is at the core for many alternative therapies. The acid/alkaline diets purpose is to oxygenate the body and cellular fluids by raising the body pH. The Ozone therapy protocol increases the oxygen dynamic within the body. Oxygen is the key and the most vital factor in everything that sustains robust and vibrant health.

Many of Dr. Budwig's discoveries were suppressed by big business. Her discoveries of the harmful effects of margarine and other hydrogenated oils were met with fierce opposition. Those with a financial tie to the business and marketing of these hydrogenated oils made sure she was unable to continue her research, and made sure she was banned from publishing her findings in any of the scientific or medically based research journals. As long as nobody found out about her discoveries they were safe. Fortunately, some people just can't keep a secret.

The only comfort we have is that one day these same, unethical, cold blooded people will one day stand before God and have to make account for this twisted and ill fated travesty of greed and deception. How can they sleep? I guess it's not an issue when you don't have a conscience.

So goes the story of just about all suppressed, alternative cancer therapies. It's all the same everywhere. You can't put life ahead of the almighty wallet no matter who is suffering. Far too many people put their lust for that new home on the hill and a Jag in the drive over a simpler life and a clear, unpolluted, heartfelt sentiment.

The recipe calls for preferably organic, low fat cottage cheese and unrefined, virgin, cold-pressed flaxseed oil. How much or how little you use will be different and adjusted according to the severity of your condition. The average dose is 1 tablespoon of flaxseed oil to ¼ cup of cottage cheese. This can be repeated twice daily or maybe 3 times daily depending on your condition. Mix it fresh each time if possible.

Those with more advanced cancers or more serious illnesses can increase to 3 -6 tablespoons of flaxseed oil and ½ to 1 cup cottage cheese a couple of times a day. It is extremely important to mix the flaxseed oil and cottage cheese in some sort of blender or other electrical device to thoroughly bind and blend the oil with the sulfur based protein, (cottage cheese).

It must be mixed briskly to bond the molecules together. You can add honey or other fruits to the mixture to make it more palatable. Consume this mixture throughout the day, everyday.

You may want to see how your body is affected by the flaxseed oil and cottage cheese before increasing to a higher dose. See if it causes loose stools or anything uncomfortable. It should be fine but as always it is best to start slow and monitor your tolerance levels.

You can always slowly work up to a higher dose. Once you get there you can stay there for a few weeks or a few months depending on how you are improving. If you are satisfied with the results you can then determine whether or not to reduce down a bit or not. Again it will all depend on your situation.

As with the majority of other therapies, you will achieve the most benefit if you remove all refined sugars and manufactured foods from your diet and anything hydrogenated for starters. Remember the main reason for this protocol is to remove and rebuild your current cellular metabolism.

You need to stay away from anything processed, refined or full of preservatives and chemicals. Juicing is also an important part of healing with this protocol. Eat an 80/20 diet ratio, 80% raw or in juices and 20% lightly cooked and remember to thoroughly chew your food. Give your digestive system a break anywhere and everywhere you can.

No butter, no cured, deli style foodstuffs, no meat or animal fats (especially meats that contain preservatives, hormones, chemicals, antibiotics or are grain fed), no commercial salad dressings including, mayonnaise and any other animal based concoction. No dairy products either with the obvious exception of the cottage cheese.

Always buy your flaxseed oil in a dark colored, refrigerated, opaque container and keep it refrigerated after opening. It is best to buy the oil and not the capsules just for the sake of freshness. Dr. budwig advised against buying flaxseeds whole and then grinding them. They can lose their potency in as little as 10-15 minutes. You also get a better bond blending with the cottage cheese using the oil. Make sure you mix the ingredients together for at least 40-60 seconds to achieve maximum binding of the oil and cottage cheese.

Dr. Budwig also advised that anyone using this specific protocol for whatever reason, stay on it for 3-5 years depending on the severity of their affliction and overall condition of health. You might also take into consideration how much and how long you have been consuming refined, adulterated, hydrogenated oils and how corrupt your cellular biology may be.

It may make more sense to stay the course for as long as is necessary as you follow its progression and remission, then adjust to a daily maintenance dose. After awhile, adjust to a maintenance dose that is manageable and reasonable for you. That could turn into a couple of times a week. It's all about your specific condition. Hopefully you will be able to monitor your progress and your blood markers through your primary care physician.

There are many testimonials of recoveries from all forms of cancer using this protocol. There are even websites devoted to this form of treatment. You can find several websites yourself for those of you that doubt such a simplistic approach. Do a Google search for flax-seed oil and cottage cheese forums. There are several where you will be able to hear firsthand accounts and experiences.

This Flaxseed Oil and Cottage Cheese Diet is also a part of the Cellect-Budwig Cancer Protocol. There is a chapter in this book that has information on the complete protocol, it is titled Cellect/ Budwig Protocol. The chapter will inform you of the Cellect portion of the protocol.

Also, although many will debate this issue, you need to spend some time out in the sunshine. Dr Budwig found that after she treated patients and had them spend some time in the sun, they felt better and more energized. Dr. Budwig stated that the sun has a stimulating effect on the liver, kidneys, gall bladder, pancreas, bladder and salivary glands.

All matter has its own vibration, as do our bodies. The sun's energy stimulates that vibration. The sun heals the mind, the body, and all it's corresponding components. Dr. Budwig tells us that after 2-3 days on her therapy your body will tolerate the sun very well. With the proper essential fats finding their way where they need to be, 20-30 minutes here and there should do the job.

In fact it will re-stimulate and re-energize your vitality and vigor. Man acts as an antenna for the sun. This interplay of photons in the sunbeams and the electrons in our foods and oils governs all the vital, life sustaining functions of the body. Did you really think that the sun was just a glorified light bulb and a heating lamp? The sun is alive and it was created to keep us alive, remember that carefully orchestrated dance, it's time to put your dancing shoes on and say hello to the sun. NO sunscreen!!!

Sunscreen contains chemicals known to cause cancer. Just limit your time in the sun to a reasonable amount and toss the protective chemical coating.

Cancer is the number 1 feared affliction of our time. The hardest part for most of us is believing the possibility that something natural defeating this affliction even exists, but exist it does. We have to believe.

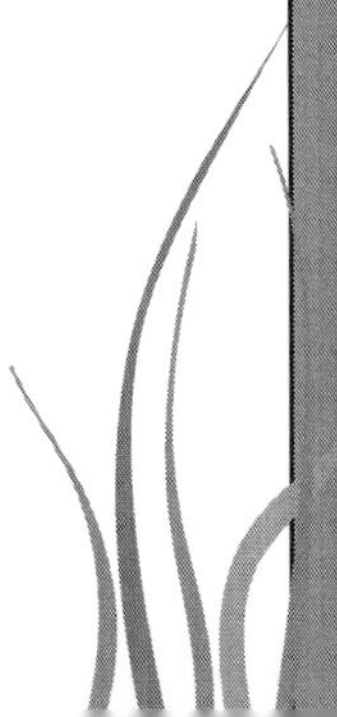

Chapter 21

Bob Wright Protocol

...MSM/LIPH...

...Phase 1...

This protocol should not be used with any of the other alkaline protocols, to much alkalinity can cause alkalosis. The protocol involves 2 distinct and consecutive phases. The MSM/LIPH is the first phase of the protocol.

The other part and second phase of this protocol involves drinking 11.5 pH alkaline water using the Kangen water system manufactured by Enagic. This device is quite expensive, running around $4,000 dollars, but well worth the investment.

The Kangen water has proven to be a very effective cancer treatment all by itself even for very fast spreading, advanced cancers. Another aspect of the protocol involves taking the "Now" nutritional supplement made by Reliv.

The MSM/LIPH purpose is to get rid of as many microbes as possible in the bloodstream. This phase of the protocol lasts for 2 weeks but is highly recommended to continue the therapy indefinitely. It is typically, later on, reduced to a reasonable maintenance dose. This would depend on the severity of your condition and how aggressive your particular type of cancer is.

It is really important to follow this protocol in order. The reason why the alkaline water is introduced later in the therapy is to prevent the cancer microbes from going into hibernation. If the pH of the cell is elevated to rapidly the cancer microbe will go into a hibernation phase and appear to be normal. This is not beneficial. Many patients believe they are cured only to find their cancer to return. The step by step process of this protocol and the strategy is to destroy microbes in the blood first using an anti-microbial substance.

Without going into too much detail, starting off with the MSM/ LIPH therapy will kill microbes in the blood. It's important to target the microbes in the blood first.

MSM

The MSM needs to be purchased from a reputable vendor to be sure you are getting pure organic sulfur. Anyone who has ever heard of this therapy knows it as the MSM/LIPH therapy. MSM is methyl-sulfonal-methane. Authentic MSM should be pure organic sulfur and that is what is required for this protocol. Many of the commercial products contain a thinned out version of what pure MSM should be.

The basic premise of this protocol is to get a sizable amount of oxygen and other microbe killing substances inside of the cancer cell and the blood. This will typically revert the cancerous cells into normal healthy cells. This also benefits healthy cells as it increases substantially, the amount of oxygen available.

The organic sulfur increases the amount of oxygen by capturing and grabbing onto the oxygen from the water and transporting it to the cells. The air we breathe is around 21% oxygen depending on where you live, oxygen in water is around 89% oxygen. This oxygen helps to increase energy production within the cell. It is important not to drink alkaline water during the first phase of this treatment. That comes in phase 2.

The best and the easiest way to administer the organic sulfur is to mix 12 tablespoons of the organic sulfur into a 1 gallon glass container of high quality, purified water. Not alkaline water, just a good quality purified water. It is imperative that the water have no trace of chlorine whatsoever. The chlorine can neutralize the effects of the organic sulfur.

The recommended dosage would be 12 ounces of this mixture twice a day. That would be the equivalent of taking 1 tablespoon twice a day without the water.

There have even been reports of the organic sulfur increasing the effectiveness of many chemotherapy drugs and that it also helps to lessen the amount of cellular damage from the chemotherapy.

It is only common sense to speak with your physician and or your pharmacist about taking the organic sulfur and whether or not there is any problem mixing with any of the other prescription medications you are taking, including chemotherapy. The dosage while on chemo would be increased by 1 tablespoon 3 times a day or 3 twelve ounce glasses of the diluted mixture 3 times a day.

The organic sulfur will also help with pain and inflammation. It also benefits and assists in the removal of toxic debris and heavy metals. It has reportedly helped to clear moderate confusion and brain fogs due to Herxheimers.

LIPH

The addition of the LIPH is a great benefit as the 2 very nicely complement one another. It's like icing on the cake. LIPH by itself has the potential to kill a wide variety of bacterial diseases, including some of the most virulent bacterial diseases such as MRSA.

The actual name of the product is known as "Alkaline Mineral Supplement Concentrate," "Alkaline Concentrate," and "Liph Immune Boosting Concentrate."

This liquid is a concentrate that comes in a 2.5 ounce bottle. It must be diluted into a 1 gallon plastic container of distilled or a high quality purified water. It should not be glass as with the organic sulfur. The silica in the glass may bind to and disrupt the action of the LIPH.

To make the diluted LIPH. Pour the entire 2.5 ounce bottle of LIPH into a 1 gallon plastic container. Fill the rest up with distilled or a good quality purified water.

The administration or dosage of the LIPH is always taken from the diluted 1 gallon plastic container. This protocol starts with 3-4 days of the organic sulfur, diluted as described above. After 3-4 days taking the 12 ounces of diluted organic sulfer twice a day, you can start taking the diluted LIPH water.

The amount of LIPH calls for 4 tablespoons or 2 ounces of the diluted LIPH solution each time you administer or take the 12 ounces of organic sulfur. This is also taken twice a day. That would be a total of 4 ounces of the LIPH diluted water and 24 ounces of the diluted organic sulfur water. This would be total for the day, being that they are taken twice daily.

Do not eat or drink anything in the hour before and after administration of these 2 protocols. You can take them together or at least within 15 minutes of one another.

Both of these supplements work by feeding the cells in your body the oxygen they need to destroy cancerous microbes. They do this through the oxygen saturated in the water.

It is important to drink plenty of water while on this protocol. You just need to stay away from any water that may be tainted with chlorine. Typically 5-8 twelve ounce glasses of a quality, micro-clustered, purified water daily will be sufficient. Remember to spread out your water intake throughout the day.

Remember the MSM/LIPH is the first phase of this protocol and is taken for 2 weeks before starting the second phase.

...Phase II...

Kangen Water

The 2nd phase introduces the high pH Kangen water. The amount of Kangen water consumed needs to be figured out by how much you weigh. The conversion is ¾ of an ounce of Kangen water per pound of body weight up to a gallon. 1 gallon of the Kangen water a day is the maximum.

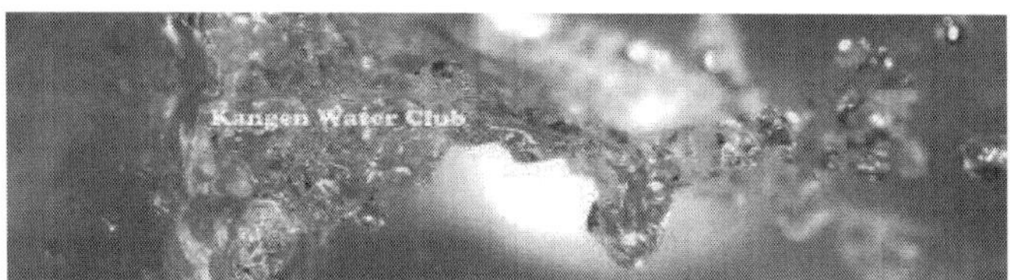

It is very important to follow the outline and steps in specific order for this protocol. You should not have to do a build-up using the Kangen water. You should be able to start on the full amount of water as the majority of the microbes in the bloodstream should be dead or very close to it.

Following phase 1 should have helped to prevent any herxheimer reaction or brain fog. If by chance it creates any herxheimers, it should be mild. Just remember to spread out your intake of water throughout the day. You can read more about what the herxheimer reaction is all about below this chapter.

The Kangen water phase should be continued for at least 3-4 months but can be continued indefinitely. It all depends on the severity of the cancer or other affliction you are dealing with and the results you experience using this protocol. Back to the being sensible thing again.

Special Note: There are several studies linking chlorinated water with cancer. Just a reminder to be sure and avoid anything that may be corrupted with chlorine, especially your water. Keep it away from your pets also.

...Lugol's Iodine Solution...

"Sunshine & Real Salt"

It is also important to get out in the sun for about 30 minutes a day, preferably not during peak UV hours. Make sure you have ample skin exposure. At the minimum your bare face and bare arms.

There is also a product called "Real Salt." This salt contains a large quantity of essential minerals which will help to facilitate oxygen transport. You can either use this salt or the one recommended in the chapter on salt. That salt is the Himilayan Pink Crystal Salt. The protocol also calls for 1-2 drops of "5% Lugol's Iodine Solution" once a day, diluted into a teaspoon of apple cider vinegar.

Iodine is crucial for the proper functioning of your thyroid gland. Once again it is our mineral depleted soils that are responsible for our iodine deficiency. Chlorine in our drinking water also displaces iodine. It all has to do with their atomic weight values, but we don't need to get into that.

Iodine has been shown to resist and help block radiation. All the blood in the body passes through the thyroid gland every 17 minutes. The thyroid gland utilizes iodine to destroy and weaken germs traveling through the bloodstream.

Iodine contributes greatly to thyroid hormone production. These hormones help to regulate our BMR (basal metabolic rate). They are also needed for the condition of our hair, nails, teeth, skin, protein synthesis, cholesterol synthesis, carbohydrate absorption, reproduction, nerve and bone formation and our everyday growth and development.

Iodine deficiency is also associated with low energy levels, nervous tension, irritability, fatigue, restlessness and other stress related disorders. It also helps to clear that occasional brain fog. It has shown great benefit in calming a hyperactive child in as little as 2-3 hours. Approximately 1 drop of 5% Lugol's Iodine mixed into a little bit of juice is usually sufficient for a younger child.

One of the biggest reasons many of us are iodine deficient, besides our mineral deficient soils, is the displacement of iodine by chlorine. Many afflictions in the body are attributed to elevated or low thyroid function or no thyroid function at all. Iodine is absolutely crucial for the proper functioning of this gland. Far too many of us have impaired thyroid function due to chlorine displacement and contamination.

Iodine deficiency has been attributed to certain types of cancer as well including, the breast, uterus and ovaries. Low iodine levels may also contribute to fibrocystic breast problems. The theory is based on the absence of iodine rendering the breast tissue more sensitive to oestrogen stimulation, producing excess secretions and creating hardening of the tissue from deposits of fibrin, similar to scar tissue. This can lead to small cysts and fibrosis.

There are 2 different ways you can administer Lugol's iodine solution. In a drink mixed with some juice or externally. Choose one or the other, not both.

If you choose to apply it externally you can apply it to the abdomen or your upper thigh. The idea of using it externally is that you will be able to tell how much your body may be lacking or deficient. Apply in a 2-3 inch patch and monitor how quickly your body absorbs the iodine. Check it every couple of hours. If your skin is clear or nearly clear after 2-4 hours you can bet that you have a deficiency problem. If it does not clear after 24 hours chances are you do not have a deficiency problem.

When taken internally with a drink, 1-2 drops is usually sufficient, depending on your weight. Sip slowly throughout and with a meal. When your body is sufficiently saturated with the iodine taken internally, you will notice within a couple of hours after taking it a release of moisture from the nose. If this occurs wait approximately 1 month and you can check again. This can typically occur after taking it for a week or 2, depending on your deficiency levels.

Same with the external application. When the iodine is no longer showing absorption and you still have a slightly faded color after 24 hours, stop the application for approximately a month and test again. Please inform your doctor before beginning any type of treatment.

Wouldn't it be nice if a lot of the symptoms you are experiencing were simply remedied by replenishing your thyroid with sufficient iodine? The thyroid is a key player in hormone production and other bodily processes. Regardless, it would be nice to know if you are deficient or not, right?

...Reliv Nutritional Supplement...

This is a nutritional support product for the MSM/LIPH part of the protocol. The protocol calls for the "Now" brand of Reliv which can be found online http://www.reliv.com/ or just go to www.reliv.com

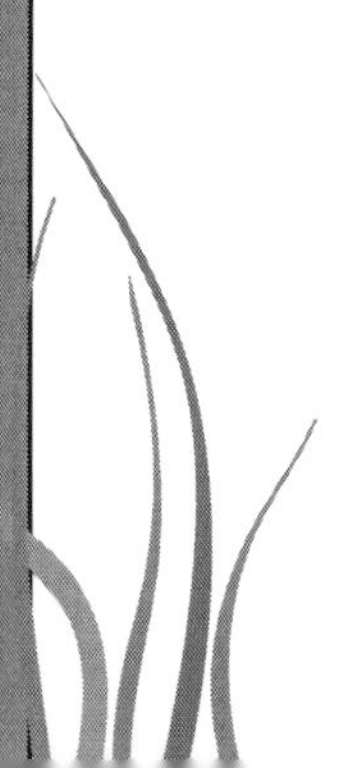

Chapter 22

Graviola

Graviola is an herb that typically grows in the rainforests. It is indigenous to warm tropical climates in North and South America. The fruit is more commonly known as Guanabana where it is sold in the local marketplace.

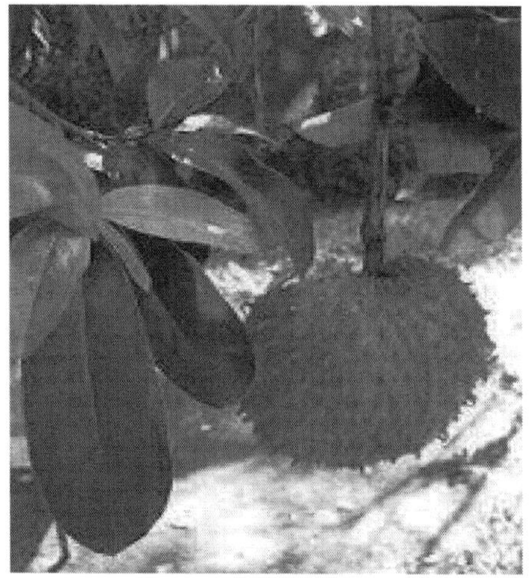

It has many medicinal and nutritional benefits. Graviola has been used for the eradication of parasites, worms, head lice, fever, gastro-intestinal disorders and also as a sedative and nervine. In many cultures it is used for inflammation, heart conditions, arthritis, difficulties in child birth, asthma, liver disorders, hypertension, depression and more. I think it comes down to that whole food, fruit deal that's supposed to be a part of our daily diet.

In research studies it has shown remarkable success against many forms of cancer. The majority of the research has centered around active compounds and chemicals in Graviola called Annonaceous acetogenins. Graviola produces these compounds in its leaves, stems, bark and fruit seeds. That doesn't mean the rest of the fruit is worthless, Ok.

This family of compounds and chemicals have been documented with anti-tumor, anti-parasitic, insecticidal and anti-microbial properties. The studies have shown it inhibits an enzyme process found only in cancerous cells. This is part of the reason why they are toxic to cancer cells but have shown no detrimental effect on healthy, non-cancerous cells.

Graviola has also shown to be effective against tumors that have not responded to conventional anti-cancer drugs (chemotherapy) and has actually shown an affinity for these unresponsive cancer cells. Without going into the highly technical aspects of this phenomena, the compounds in Graviola are sometimes able to eradicate tumors that multiple chemotherapy drugs failed to destroy.

The pharmaceutical companies are trying to figure out a way to chemically alter and synthesize the compounds in Graviola so they can patent it. Then they will market it back to you with a fancy name and a prescription. They are so incredibly clever and we are so incredibly naïve. I would just as soon consume it from the source in it's whole, unadulterated, original package.

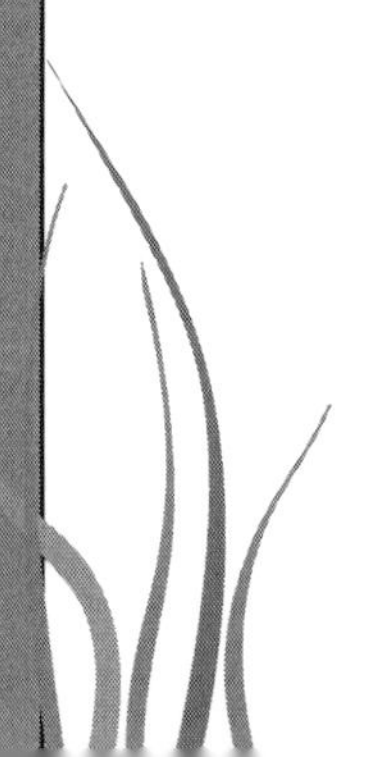

Chapter 23

Possible Cancer Side Effect Issues

...Herxheimer Reaction...

The Herxheimer reaction is a condition brought about by destroying massive amounts of cancer microbes in the body too quickly. This creates what is known as brain fog. People using any type of alternative treatment need to be aware of this phenomena. Many patients stop their alternative treatment because of this somewhat frightening side effect. It is not dangerous and is only temporary, so please do not quit your treatment.

When these microbes are destroyed they release mycotoxins into the bloodstream. These mycotoxins create a highly acidic environment causing a disruption in the clarity of radio signals the brain uses to communicate.

This temporary brain fog can be pretty intense and severe. Many patients really believe they are brain dead. Fortunately, there is a way to avoid this reaction.

The trick is to slowly build up to the recommended dosage amount. If the recommended dosage is hypothetically, 2 ounces at a time, twice a day and 6 hours apart, start with a lower dosage. This is what is called a build up phase to the treatment. I spoke about this before in a previous chapter. It's about taking baby steps as long as you have the luxury of time.

This is the one of the best ways to avoid the Herxheimer reaction. If the dosage calls for 2 ounces, twice a day, 6 hours apart, start with maybe a half ounce, 2 times a day, 6 hours apart. Monitor how you feel. Maybe you do this for 2-3 days and see how your body is handling this amount.

If you are having only moderate to no reactions, move up to 1 ounce, 2 times a day 6 hours apart and see how you feel. Just understand that you are hopefully destroying cancer cells and that the process can produce some uncomfortable symptoms. Be aware and adjust from there.

If you are dealing with one of the electro-medicine devices and it recommends 2 hours of the electrification and 2 hours with a magnetic pulser than adjust your time accordingly. Start with 20 minutes of electrification and 20 minutes with the magnetic pulser for a few days.

With the electrification you can also adjust the intensity of the current. Start out on a lower intensity and gradually increase. See how you feel. Same with the ozonated water. If it calls for 3-6 glasses of ozonated water daily, start with 1 a day. Same with any of the other protocols, do a build up and monitor your symptoms. As a general rule, most alternative medical practitioners recommend an average 5 day build up phase to avoid the Herxheimer reaction.

If you are attempting a protocol that has very little information on its use then they recommend an even longer build up. Kind of like being stranded somewhere strange and your not sure what is edible and what might keep you alive. You nibble a tiny little bit of something that looks promising just in case it is a poison. Find out if it will kill you before you decide to make a meal of it.

It would also be a good idea to do your own research, especially if you are treating or dealing with something other than cancer. Find out what type of organisms you may be killing off, what type of symptoms you might experience and what type of microbes or pathogens you will be targeting. That way you can get a little better idea of what to expect as far as potential side effects.

Number 1, just be aware that any brain fog you may experience has a name, (Herxheimer reaction), and that it is a temporary and fully recoverable side effect. It will go away, you are not losing your mind. The positive side of this condition is that it generally means your therapy is working.

...Cachexia...

The Cachexia cycle is the wasting away of the body. It is a vicious and life stealing cycle for the cancer patient. As long as the cancer is thriving, surviving, and continues to grow unabated, the cachexia cycle will continue to slowly but surely reduce the patient to a sad and frail image of their former self.

Cachexia is defined by a loss of body mass even for patients that are consuming a reasonable amount of calories. Cachexia severely weakens the patient typically resulting in a loss of appetite, anemia, loss of energy, progressive loss of weight and muscle atrophy.

Cachexia is a very serious condition that needs to be addressed. Statistics show that between 20-40% of cancer deaths are directly related and caused by cachexia. As of now there are very limited conventional treatments available for cancer cachexia. Pharmaceutical appetite stimulants and nutrient supplementation have had very limited effects.

Therapeutic studies continue with the use of pharmaceutical drugs and supplementation. The use of multitargeted therapies seems to have the most success for now. Conventional studies continue.

Cachexia manifests because of the way the anaerobic cancer cell receives its energy, through the fermentation of sugar (glucose), instead of the uptake of oxygen as in a healthy cell. The cancer cell incompletely metabolizes glucose with lactic acid as a by-product. When this lactic acid finds its way back into the bloodstream, it travels through the liver where it is converted back into glucose. The whole process expends an enormous amount of valuable energy.

This unconventional and inefficient pathway of energy metabolism yields only 2 moles of ATP (adenosine triphosphate) energy per mole of glucose compared to 38 moles of ATP performed by a normal healthy cell. That's a big difference. One of the reasons it is called a wasting disease. The cancer cell is only utilizing about 5% of the available energy (2 moles compared to 38 moles) so in turn it is "wasting" available energy.

Too many die from malnutrition well before the cancer finishes the job. I know the cancer initiated the malnutrition, it's just sad that more emphasis is not put into regulating or addressing this horrendous and viscous cycle.

The cancer, if left unchecked, continues this barbaric cycle. The body slowly wastes away, expending enormous amounts of energy trying to keep the cancer cells well nourished. Not only does this constant and continuous cycle of converting lactic acid back into glucose exert a tremendous amount of energy, this lactic acid lowers the pH of the body and creates an ideal and acid filled environment for the cancer to thrive and proliferate.

As the appetite decreases with the body not receiving the nourishment that it needs, it will start breaking down fat stores and proteins. A normal, oxygen rich, healthy cell, metabolizes 15 times more efficiently than an anaerobic cancer cell. The cancer cell metabolizes through the inefficient process of fermentation. This increases the cancer cells need for even more sugar, hindering the amount of available sugars for normal, healthy cell, energy production.

There is an alternative treatment that deals directly with cachexia. "Hydrazine Sulphate blocks a key enzyme in the liver that allows lactic acid to be converted into glucose." Thus shutting down the cycle.

Before considering the use of hydrazine sulphate, a person must make drastic changes to their diet. They must stop feeding the cancer where and when they are able. Next, you need to understand and know that just because a cancer patient starts losing weight does not necessarily mean they are suffering from cachexia.

Any drastic dietary change will typically involve some weight loss. Just be sure that you take that into consideration before diagnosing cachexia and the possible administration and use of hydrazine sulphate.

A lot of it will depend on how the patient feels. Are they sick all the time? Is their appetite gone? Are they coherent? Is their energy level depleted? Remember that cancer cells have to eat and they will literally eat the person's body if they have too.

Hydrazine sulphate, "interrupts the ability of the liver to convert lactic acid from tumors into glucose. This helps to starve the tumors and inhibits their ability to metastasize."

A Dr. Joseph Gold studied the chemical process of glycogenisis. He determined that if he inhibited the PEP CK enzyme, he could interrupt this process. He discovered hydrazine sulphate, a substance that is made very inexpensively, is simple to use, fuels military rockets and is able to shrink tumors.

In his early studies with animals, Dr. Gold discovered that in greater than 50% of the animals he tested with cancer, he was able to stop the process of glycogenisis, stop the cachexia cycle, and the animals began gaining weight. With the sugars cut off to the tumors, the tumors began to shrink.

Hydrazine Sulphate has a lot of warnings, drug interactions and foods that need to be avoided containing the amino acid tyramine. If someone is suffering from severe cachexia it would be a good idea to look into hydrazine sulphate further. http://www.cancertutor.com/Cancer/Hydrazine.html to go to a website that will be able to give you more information on foods to avoid.

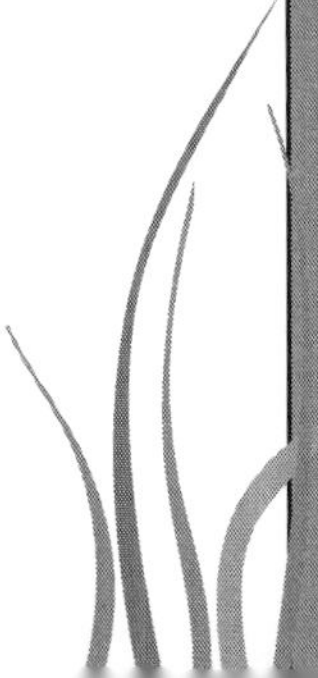

Chapter 24

Dental Issue's Interfering With Treatments

There are several things that need to be addressed after an initial cancer diagnosis. Before you decide on what course of treatment to pursue, you need to try and figure out what may have contributed to its occurrence in the first place and remove any and all potentials. Any and all that are within your control.

Were there any warning signals? What was your body telling you? What symptoms were you experiencing? What other health related issue's were you dealing with and how long were you dealing with them? Is there any reason to believe they could have played a role in the development of this disease??? If so, they need to be addressed, removed and dealt with immediately.

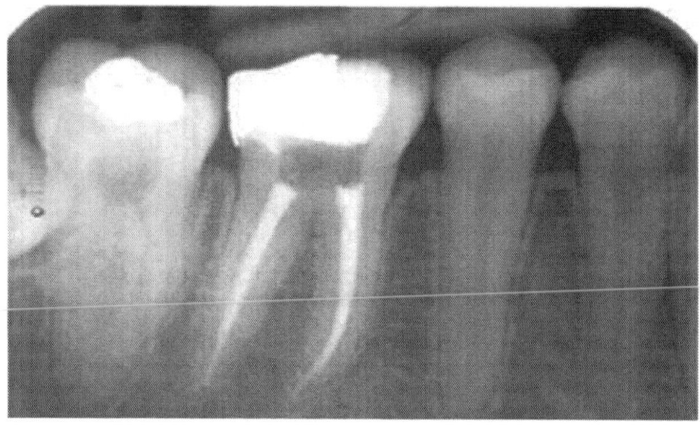

Believe it or not your teeth can have a profound impact on your health, the development of the cancer and the efficacy of the treatment you choose to pursue. Toxic teeth have been confirmed as an issue that needs to be addressed when dealing with a diagnosis as serious as cancer or anything else for that matter.

One of the primary dental issue's that needs to be taken into consideration is silver fillings. Although it is not used quite as extensively today, anyone who still has these toxic fillings in their mouth needs to have them removed post haste. Many of us, depending on our age, still have these toxic amalgams in our mouths.

In order to make these silver fillings more pliable, and the reason it is called an amalgam is that the silver is usually mixed or blended with mercury. Many of these amalgams are over 50% mercury. The vapor alone is extremely toxic seeing that mercury is one of the most toxic substances known to man.

Doesn't it seem odd that the directions given to dentists along with this toxic amalgam are to never, ever, ever touch it with your fingers, and certainly do not leave it lying out and about because of the potential of inhaling any toxic vapors.

They even have very strict protocols for disposal of this toxic substance. Of course they still considered it Ok to put in your mouth. Wow, really? I could use some really choice words right now and it's really hard not to considering the insanity of it all, and the massive suffering created by this unfathomable travesty on our health. OMG!

The dentists that had a conscience refused to continue using this common practice and started using other materials whenever they could. Even though they knew the dangers of this commonly used amalgam, they were required to keep its potential for harm to themselves or, risk losing their medical licenses. It was a well known fact that just breathing the vapors could cause brain damage.

They had more than theorized that mercury amalgam fillings could be tied to illnesses such as Parkinsons, Alzheimers, MS and many degenerative forms of arthritis. The greatest proof they had was when these type fillings were removed and replaced, the condition of their patients greatly improved or, their conditions went away altogether. It was way past being coincidence.

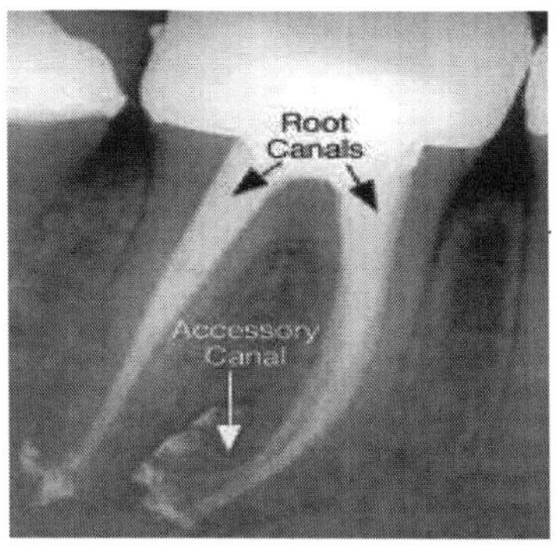

A Dr. Eggleston from USC ran a test on T-lymphocyte levels on a patient with mercury amalgam fillings. Since it was supposed that the presence of mercury fillings had a direct impact on the quality and health of the immune system, a T-lymphocyte test might prove the theory beyond a reasonable doubt.

In a healthy immune system, T-lymphocytes typically comprise up to 80% of a normal, healthy patients immune system. The woman used in the study had a T-lymphocyte level of 47% prior to the removal of the mercury fillings. After removal of the mercury fillings her T-lymphocyte levels rose to 73%. This drastic improvement supported his theory and lay firm his suspicions.

Several other tests and procedures have been performed proving that mercury amalgams do pose a more than significant risk to the body and our health. Quite surprisingly, even to the extent of causing spontaneous remission of some cancers.

Seems a bit odd and very coincidental that the first reported cases of Hodgkins disease occurred soon after mercury fillings first appeared on the market.

Several European countries have banned the use of mercury amalgam fillings. Many people fortunately have a strong enough immune system to fight off some of the ill effects of mercury toxicity. Those in the grip of any serious illness or disease are strongly advised to have them removed. Even if you are not currently suffering from any type of infirmity, if they're in your mouth they need to not be.

Removal of these toxic fillings should only be performed by a qualified biological dentist. Improper removal can cause major health related issue's so, do not trust your health or your mouth in the hands of anyone other than a well qualified and experienced practitioner.

There are times and circumstances when you will need to find a dentist even more experienced, even more qualified than a biological dentist. A specialist in treating long term infections or caries in the mouth. This is vitally and undeniably beyond a reasonable doubt, extremely critical. These long term, deeply imbedded infections from root canals and extractions are a major cause of cancer. It is not just hearsay, this is fact. Don't leave it to chance, please don't leave it to chance, chance is not your friend.

Another dental issue of great concern if you are dealing with cancer is root canals. Although root canals seem to be the perfect answer to a damaged tooth, being that you are able to keep the tooth for eating and smiling purposes, they can cause extreme consequences. Many dentists will tell you differently and many will even laugh in your face. It's your choice, the research is pretty convincing and being embarrassed by your dentist is nothing compared to your life.

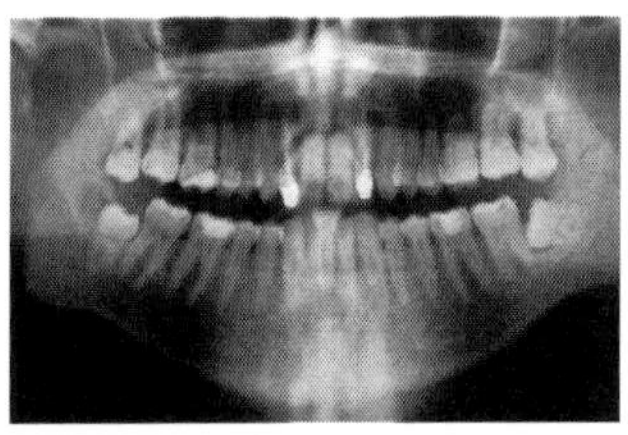

The tissue and blood vessels that would normally bring nutrients to that area have been removed, leaving what's left susceptible to infection. This is extremely difficult to treat being that there is an extensive network of tiny tubules.

These tubules are microscopic and very difficult for any antibiotic or any bacterial to reach. Any bacteria can morph from aerobic (oxygenated) to anaerobic (without oxygen). This form of bacteria can leach into the surrounding tissue and eventually find its way into the bloodstream where it will progress throughout the entire body becoming systemic. This is where major health related issue's are born.

Early in the 1900's a Dr. Weston Price set out to research and prove the dangers of root canal filled teeth. It is only recently that a Dr. George F. Meinig condensed Dr. Price's original 1,174 pages of research and put it into a user friendly book called "The Root Canal Cover-Up."

He was the perfect candidate for this effort being that he was one of the founding members of the American Association of Endodontists, root canal specialists. Apparently Dr. Meinig and other researchers agreed that no matter how well done and how thoroughly sterilized a root canal, they can never reach all of the infected areas.

A very detailed and disturbing test conducted by Dr. Price confirmed these suspicions. He took a small portion of an extracted root canal from a heart attack patient and placed that small portion under the skin of a living rabbit. Within 10 days that particular rabbit died of a heart attack. He then removed that same piece of tooth from the dead rabbit and again placed that same piece under the skin of another rabbit, same results.

He did this over and over again with the same results. The rabbit would die within about 10 days, removing the speculation of coincidence. He found that whatever the affliction, heart disease, arthritis, kidney disease etc. the rabbit would assume the same malady. He did this with a root canaled tooth from a woman with crippling arthritis, within 48 hours the rabbit acquired the same severe, crippling arthritis.

Amazingly, after this woman had her root canaled tooth extracted, her arthritic symptoms improved dramatically. To further quiet the critics, he placed a small, perfectly healthy tooth under the skin of a rabbit with no abnormal effects whatsoever. Hmmmmm

The main reason for including this information in the book is that it can be a very serious threat to your health and the strength of your immune system. These issue's can also greatly reduce the effectiveness of any therapy you decide upon. This information is mostly ignored or unheard of by the mainstream dental authorities.

A Dr. Josef Issels from Germany who specialized in the treatment of cancer said that 90% of his cancer patients had root canal filled teeth in their mouths. Before starting treatment he required that all his patients have any root canal procedures removed. He incredibly has the highest remission rate of any cancer doctor for late stage cancers.

In Dr. Issels book, "Cancer—A Second Opinion" he states that the thioethers, the poison created by bacteria living in the absence of oxygen, have all the components necessary to create spontaneous cancers in man.

He conducted further tests with infrared emissions. These emissions were present around the area of a root canaled tooth. A tumor also emitted these infrared emissions.

In one of his cancer patients, after the root canaled tooth was extracted, these emissions decreased while at the same time the emissions from the tumor also decreased. The evidence is quite compelling and questionably frightening. You need to take this under extreme consideration and take whatever action necessary.

If you think you are safe by having porcelain crowns in your mouth, you might be surprised to know that between 50-75% of crowns, including porcelain crowns, contain nickel. With a porcelain crown the nickel is what is typically used on the inside to bond to the porcelain.

Many Dr.'s agree that although nickel is not as active as mercury it is far more carcinogenic. Nickel is generally alloyed with stainless steel. Old fashioned metal braces for teeth and some dentures are made with this alloyed pairing.

There is a report of a woman that had been diagnosed with kidney disease. The doctors treating her could not pinpoint the reason for her condition and kidney failure. They finally decided on a special method of testing and determined she was highly reactive to nickel. The doctor then asked if she had had any dental work done in the last several years.

She informed the doctor that she had 3 porcelain crowns put in her mouth within the last several years. Knowing that many of the porcelain crowns had the nickel/stainless steel alloy, he recommended she have them removed immediately and replaced. Strange days indeed, soon after their removal, all of her symptoms of kidney failure just went away and disappeared.

Another story told by a Dr. Hal Huggins, reports of a woman who had had a lumpectomy for breast cancer. She was curious about a paper she had heard about linking breast cancer and nickel alloyed, dental crowns.

She happened to be attending a support group in her area and found out about another woman who had gone to the same dentist, had the same type of crown put in, and developed the very same type of breast tumor a couple of years later.

They then investigated further and curiously found several other women who had had the same type of breast tumors and had gone to the same dentist and received the same type of nickel alloyed crowns.

It all goes back to the premise of the body functioning as a whole. When something goes awry, seek the cause, do not become complacent by covering up and managing the symptoms with prescription medications. That is not a reasonable option anymore. Something caused and created this breakdown, find it, treat it, fix it, remove it and kill it. Give your body the chance to perform.

When you ask your dentist if there is a possibility of nickel in any of your crowns, most will reply that they are stainless steel and porcelain. If they do contain stainless steel they are generally alloyed with another metal. It would be nice to nail down whether or not that alloy is nickel and whether or not you need to be concerned.

If there is any chance of a toxic metal imbedded in your mouth it would be highly recommended to contact the proper, biological dentist and have them professionally removed and replaced with an appropriate alternative. It could have a drastic effect on the quality of your health and the effectiveness of any decided upon treatment.

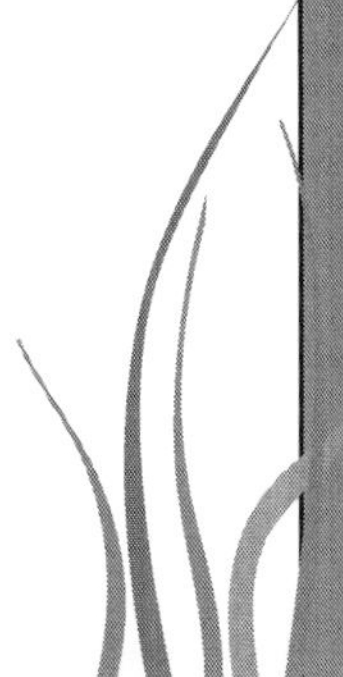

Chapter 25

The Diet

The cancer diet is crucial no matter what alternative treatment or treatments you decide upon. Defeating your cancer goes beyond the treatment itself. If you are not eating cancer defeating, immune stimulating foodstuffs than you are more or less adding unnecessary fuel to an already out of control fire.

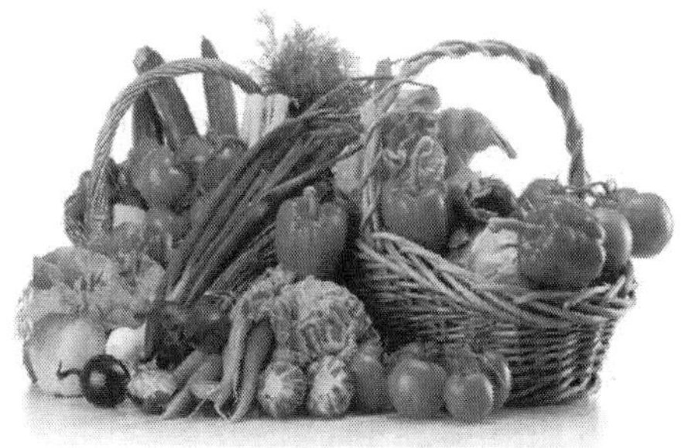

Many patients have cured their afflictions using only a massive dietary change in their eating habits. Your diet is very powerful. If you had been eating a well balanced, organic, 80% raw, additive free diet in the first place, cancer more than likely would never have reared its less than attractive profile.

But that didn't happen, we generally trust the integrity of our protective government institutions and our food suppliers. The majority of us trust the world that nothing so damning and destructive to our bodies would ever have been offered up for public consumption, oops, our bad.

Without exaggerating, the diet you choose while initiating your therapy can make or break its chances for success. The diet must compliment the therapy, it must work synergistically by strengthening the power of the protocol, it's a team effort.

It will be a rough road at first because of the food you are addicted too. You may not think that this will be a problem but, just as with anything, everything wants and needs to eat, including microbes, fungi and other pathogens inside your body. They all survive on something you are putting in your mouth. Many people crave the very foods they are allergic too. When one of these pathogens needs to eat, it will send your body a strong signal to find that food source, and naturally you will more than likely comply to that request.

Different alternative cancer treatments require a different diet. There are a few basic aspects and foods that remain pretty much standard in any cancer diet, but many, depending on the protocol, restrict certain foods that may be allowed in another alternative treatment.

A lot of the foods you need to avoid during your road to recovery include; no refined sugar, no refined flour, no dairy (the exception would be the cottage cheese in the "flax-seed oil and cottage cheese protocol"), no meat, and yes chicken is meat, fish is meat and pig is meat (some of the diets do include small portions of free range, grass fed, organic meats). The idea is to stay away from anything that takes energy away from the task at hand, fighting the cancer.

The majority of meats are tainted with far too many chemicals, hormones, pesticides and antibiotics to be of any benefit. Back to the list; no soda pops, no cigarettes, no alcohol, no hydrogenated oils or deep fried foods, no artificial sweeteners (aspartame, NutraSweet, Splenda, Equal etc.), no MSG (although there are many synonyms that keep MSG very cleverly disguised), no chlorinated or fluoridated water, no microwave cooking, no aluminum pots, pans or utensils and generally stay away from any food that has been altered, rearranged, enhanced or marketed to be something it isn't. A lot is just common sense, use it!

A large proportion of your daily food intake should be raw to keep the all important enzymes intact. A small percentage of your food lightly steamed will help with the digestion of the raw portion. Cooking destroys vital enzymes if you are consuming mainly cooked foods. The enzymes your body needs to extract the nutrients and effectively complete digestion will be absent or dead. But you hopefully already knew all that from reading a previous chapter.

There are many fruits and vegetables that have very powerful cancer killing properties and our all so important enzymes. A few of these would be broccoli, cauliflower, brussel sprouts, red beets, carrots, green asparagus, cabbage, red and green peppers, jalapeno and chili peppers, spinach, kale, collard greens, romaine, tomatos, figs, watermelon, lemons, oranges, strawberries, raspberries, grapes, apples, grapefruit, papayas, apricots, bananas, avocados, blueberries etc. Ok I know that was a little more than a few but you get the idea, raw, raw, raw, I know, I sound like a cheerleader.

Like I said before, most of the alternative cancer treatments that have restricted fruits and or vegetables will include that information. The biggest one would probably be the Gerson Therapy. There are many items that we would typically include in our daily meal preps that are forbidden on the Gerson Therapy. Some are only restricted at the beginning of the protocol and then slowly re-introduced later on.

Best advice would be to consume as many raw, organic fruits and vegetables as possible. They are loaded with all the essentials and the essentials are essential. Essentially that is what I'm trying to say. Sorry for the humor, figured you might need a break.

By the way, many patients have used a carrot juice diet to cure their cancers. They would need to be organic and raw. Hopefully grown in some really rich, mineral dense soil. Several glasses a day. You may turn orange but don't worry, it will go away. Some add red beets to the mixture or an apple but the carrot juice needs to be the main attraction.

Lemons are also very beneficial to add to your diet. Fresh organic lemon juice is a great addition to most of the therapies as lemons help to alkalize the body. It is best to drink it in warm, purified water when you wake up, at least 30 minutes before anything else. Another forbidden item in the cancer diet is refined table salt. Never use table salt even if you are not sick.

Otherwise you need to remove the man enhanced foodstuffs from your diet and eat the caveman diet, minus the animals. I have a detailed article on my blog that you absolutely need to read explaining why it is crucial to remove animal based proteins from your diet. You can http://shockinghealthnewsletter.com/blog to read the article.

There are many brands of supplements and juice drinks that are very beneficial to help get some much needed nutrition and energy into the cancer patient. Tahitian Noni Juice and Xango Mangosteen Juice are 2 of the best. Also a quality green product like wheatgrass is also recommended, unless specifically advised not to. Just make sure the wheatgrass meets the standards set forth in the Wheatgrass chapter of this book.

Remember if you have or will be looking to buy a juicer you need to buy one that pulverizes the entire fruit or vegetable. This way you can include the seeds, skins, fiber and grasses into your juicing. You need the fiber! Also remember that it has its highest nutritional value right after it is made so try and drink it right away. Although don't drink it to fast or you will more than likely get a tummy ache. Swish it around with your saliva to help alkalize before you swallow. This will help avoid stomach upset.

Sprouts are also very nutritious but best grown at home. They are very easy to grow in jars at home. They sprout really fast. Just buy the seeds and let them soak in some purified water. A quart glass jar works well, soak for around 3-4 hours. Some require a little longer, drain and cover with some cheesecloth and a rubber band. The next day add some purified water and rinse them again and drain. Most of the time that will do it. Just keep an eye if they get really dry. If so, rinse again. You are now a certified sprouter.

The only nuts allowed on a cancer diet are almonds, macadamia nuts and walnuts. Cashews and peanuts are forbidden. Soy products are a bit controversial. They are typically heavily sprayed with pesticides so finding a quality organic product, pesticide free should be Ok. Probably best to stay away from any processed soy products like tofu.

Like I said before or probably several times before, your diet is just as important as the therapy. You can effectively kill the therapy simply by ingesting the wrong foodstuffs and feeding the fire within.

Your conventional doctor, so much of the time, will typically not even mention diet with you. It is astonishing the number of cancer patients I have spoken to who were never even questioned about their diet. It's usually not a focus in the curriculum or the textbooks of the conventional medical schools.

It is beyond comprehension. Do not dismiss this critical aspect, it will absolutely have to change for your condition, for your life and for the rest of your long and prosperous recovery.

...Hydrochloric Acid...

Hydrochloric acid is the only acid that our body actually produces. Any other acids are by-products of our metabolism. Hydrochloric acid is unconditionally critical for life. Hydrochloric acid is our front line of defense for any unwelcome microbes in our food. It will destroy, kill and digest these foreign entities.

It helps to clean up the metabolic by-products from our inappropriate and unacceptable food combinations. Therefore, sufficient amounts of hydrochloric acid help to reduce excess tissue acid waste in the body.

It is vital in breaking down our food since it is the first substance in the stomach that begins the process of digestion. With our over consumption of various adulterated foods, imagine the excess of harmful, metabolic, acid waste residues if our bodies are not producing enough hydrochloric acid. This is the prelude to illness and infirmity.

Hydrochloric acid maintains the proper acid/alkaline balance in our digestive tract. After it has completed this all important function it becomes alkaline. There are several vitamins, minerals and the 8 essential aminos acids that are dependent upon the presence of hydrochloric acid. It assists in absorption from the foods we eat. Improper levels block this from happening.

Hydrochloric acid levels play a very important role in the body that cannot be overlooked, especially if you are dealing with cancer or some other major affliction. When your levels of hydrochloric acid are balanced in the stomach, it initiates the measured release of secretin, an alkaline based hormone from the pancreas.

This hormone causes the pancreas to produce generous amounts of a very alkaline forming bicarbonate. These bicarbonate secretions by the pancreas create an appropriate pH for the action of our pancreatic enzymes.

When hydrochloric acid levels are too low it interferes with another hormone CCK (cholecystokinin). CCK is produced in the small intestine where it sends a signal to the gall bladder to release necessary bile. When this hormone is hindered by insufficient hydrochloric acid levels, bile output is reduced, affecting the absorption, assimilation and delivery of nutrients. This is not beneficial to your health.

The list of conditions associated with low hydrochloric acid levels is disturbing. This is an issue that is mostly ignored by conventional medicine but critical for your recovery. It plays a significant role in our body processes.

...Salt...

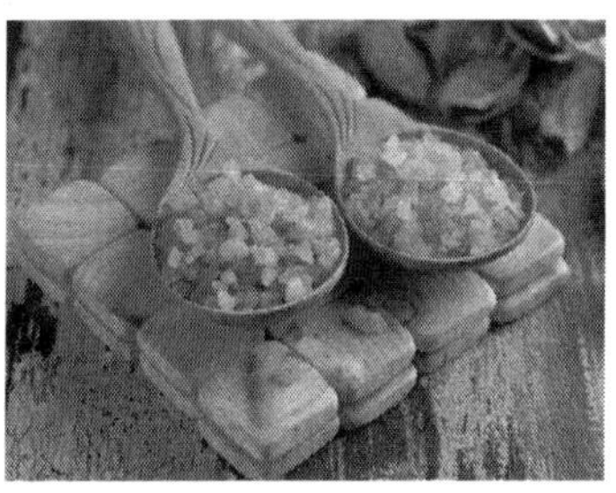

I'm not sure why salt has gotten such a bad rap in terms of health. Maybe it's just a ploy to sell more medications. Without salt we cease to function. Salt is vital to our survival. A lack of salt is a major contributor to various different afflictions including asthma, allergies and a plethora of degenerative diseases.

In times past salt was used as a trading medium similar to gold. Many different cultures knew that salt was crucial to their survival and health. It has also been used throughout antiquity as a healing medication.

Salt and potassium help to regulate the action of water in the body. Potassium keeps the water inside of the cell and salt balances the amount of water held outside of the cell. When we are dehydrated and the interior of our cells lack the proper amount of water, the body draws on the water held outside of the cell for emergency injection.

When water is unavailable inside of the cell the body will filter and inject water from outside of the cell into the cell. This is part of the reason for swelling and or edema. The body uses salt to retain and hold onto water for emergency situations. When the cell is dehydrated (lack of sufficient water) and in need of water, an increase in pressure is necessary to inject water from outside of the cell, into the cell. This is what is commonly referred to as hypertension (high blood pressure). Are you following this? Could your high blood pressure be from a chronically dehydrated condition?

The body purposely holds onto salt in its attempt to hold onto more water for emergencies. Once the cells and the body become hydrated the excess salt is eliminated in your urine. You could always consider drinking more water instead of taking the overly prescribed diuretics and other blood pressure medications.

If salt has been restricted in your diet, you need to slowly and gradually increase your water consumption. Anyone on prescription diuretics or other prescribed medications should consult with their physician beforehand. Since they are in the business of prescribing medications, you will probably need to request weening off the medication and increasing your water consumption. Once your water levels are up closer to the recommended daily amount, salt should be added back into your diet. The more water you drink the more any edema will dissipate and be eliminated.

The thing is, if you consume the proper amount of water, the body will naturally eliminate any excess salt. The right type of salt needs to be a regular part of your diet but, you can't add salt to your diet without adding the additional water.

Don't be fooled by all the brands of salt claiming to be sea salt, especially the bleached white, sea salts. Any salt at one time came from the sea. That means that any salt is actually sea salt, right? Even table salt would be processed sea salt. One of the best quality natural salts on the market is Himalayan Pink Crystal Salt. This salt contains 84 minerals and trace minerals including iodine.

Many times your bodies cries for food, or what we assume are cravings for food, are actually an attempt by the body to obtain more salt, more minerals. You know how good those salty, bad for you snack foods are. Have you ever noticed how badly some people crave salt. Their food is prepared with adequate salt and then when it's put in front of them, they add even more. Don't you think there is a message there. A message of why those salty snacks taste so good.

Our bodies are trying to tell us something. Why not give your body a full spectrum, complex and complete salt. When you feed the body the wrong type of salt (table salt), it just wants more. All of these addictive cravings making you crazy, and God forbid overweight, may just be a craving for the right kind of salt and some good quality water. Hmmmm. Something to think about.

You can't increase your water consumption without increasing your salt consumption. Salt helps to keep water in the blood and blood vessels. Salt is a vital component to nerve communication and hydroelectric energy in the body. Salt is also a very effective antihistamine and can help alleviate asthma and dry cough. Salt helps to clear excess acidity from our cells, including our brain cells.

Salt assists in maintaining muscle tone and strength. Involuntary leakage of urine and bladder control can be a sign of salt deficiency. It helps to regulate sleep patterns. A few grains of salt left on the tongue after drinking a full glass of water will help to induce deep sleep. Salt helps to clear mucous, catarrh and phlegm from the lungs and sinuses. Salt can help in the prevention of gout and other arthritic conditions. It prevents muscle cramps and is vital in maintaining strong bones.

Salt aids in the absorption of nutrients through the intestinal tract. Surprisingly, salt also helps to preserve serotonin and melatonin levels in our brain. With water and salts ability to assist in the removal of toxins from our cells, essential amino acids are spared and are able to focus on producing greater quantities of melatonin, serotonin and tryptamine. This process helps to alleviate depression, foul moods and in turn elevates a more positive self image.

There's a story of a woman that was so crippled up with arthritic pains and severely damaged knees, she was barely able to get herself up out of bed. She had heard about this book and decided to listen to Dr. Batmanghelidj's advice. The book is titled "Your Body's Many Cries For Water." Soon after implementing water and salt into her diet her symptoms began to change. She is now able to walk several blocks and she is able to go on trips without worrying about her embarrassing bladder control issue's. Such a simple concept. There's no money to be made in salt and water but what a simple thing we all should be doing.

Adjusting the amount and quality of water in your cancer therapy needs to include the proper amount and quality of salt. The 2 need to go together. They perform so many vital functions in the body.

Salt is necessary to help balance sugar levels in the blood and reduces the amount of insulin needed by diabetics. Salt in the diet also helps to maintain libido. Overall, without going into further details, let's just assume that salt is vital to a well balanced body. The right type of salt is also an important consideration.

Another point of interest. A Dr. H. Alderman and his associates, from the Albert Einstein College of Medicine published an article stating that patients on a restricted low salt diet were more likely to die of a stroke or heart attack than those who used salt liberally. Another Dr. David McCurron from the Department of Nephrology at Oregon Health Science University, Portland, stated that patients with a daily intake of calcium, magnesium and potassium had no elevated rise in blood pressure, in fact, they determined that it may even lower it.

Salt regulates the water levels outside of the cell and potassium, calcium and magnesium regulate water levels inside of the cell. These 4 elements are essential for cellular health along with water. A 1/8 to 1/4 teaspoon of naturally mineralized Himilayan

Pink Crystal salt should be taken with every 4-5 glasses of water. Your new found dietary habits and organic foods will also contribute to your daily essentials. Your whole world and outlook will change after you make the decision to employ all of these amazing yet simple health benefits.

...Tumors...

It's interesting to note that when people are diagnosed with a cancerous tumor, the urgency to have it removed immediately is overwhelming. Conventional medical doctors are consumed with tumors and the issues that go along with their revelation. They want to cut asap, this can sometimes be a fatal mistake.

Chances are this tumor has been growing for the most part, many, if not tens of years. If this tumor is unsightly or in a dangerous location where it may cause other serious issues then, removal is always something to consider, otherwise, the facts will usually speak for themselves.

The fact of the matter is that you cannot cut out cancer, you cannot remove cancer and proclaim that you are healed. Women that have their breast removed and claim they are cured is misleading. Many have the other breast removed just to be safe, really? Why? This is pure, fear induced insanity. The cause must be addressed or it will return, count on it.

What kind of a fix is that anyway? I love how removing some damaged body part is so often the decided upon option in conventional medicine. Just get rid of it and that should do it, right? Wrong, you have to figure out why it failed by working your way backwards through the maze, determining how that damage came to be. There's always a reason. There's always a process.

You don't just keep removing parts that become diseased and expect anything even close to a cure. You have to investigate the reason, you have to be a body process detective, an internal investigator. You have to find the root of the problem, the seat of the fire.

When the tumor is located in an area where it is not posing a significant health threat, the patients that opted not to have it removed surgically lived as long and sometimes lived longer than those that decided on the surgery and had it removed.

Then there's always the chance of disrupting the cancer cells and having them spread elsewhere in the body. That can be a disaster. Most doctor's know this and will advise you as to the risks. At least they should.

You need to ask your doctor why this breast or whatever became cancerous, how and why did the tumor form? What happened in my body that created the environment for this to manifest? Ask if there is any way your body can deal with this tumor without the need for surgery. Ideally, isn't this what needs to happen to prevent it from occurring somewhere else in the future? What went wrong? Don't be afraid to question all aspects of their decisions.

...Final Thoughts...

I just want to say that I am grateful and I did appreciate what seemed to be genuine concern on the part of just about all the conventional healthcare professionals we met along the way. I know they wanted to be able to help. Actually, the more I learned about all the different alternative therapies the more I felt sorry for their lack of knowledge and experience with alternative therapies.

I bet many of them knew a lot more than they were willing to mention. Of course, nothing was ever mentioned anyway. Their job could be on the line if they did. For all they knew we could be spies for the drug cartels. The only thing I couldn't get my head around was watching patients suffer and die when you knew there were obviously other, non-invasive, natural options available.

Even if they did have any knowledge they could potentially lose their actual medical license by association or by offering up what they did know. Nearly all of them sincerely wanted to help, somehow, someway. Their hands were tied by their loyalty to the conventional medical establishment and their job security in providing for their families.

What you decide is the best course of treatment for your situation is ultimately up to you. Many of the above treatments can be combined, at least parts of them can. Many of them cannot be combined. Be sure and consult with the vendor or practitioner of whichever treatment you decide upon.

You also need to take into consideration how far advanced your condition is and how much time you have or may not have before you put together a strategy.

Whatever treatment you decide on will also be affected by the type of cancer you are dealing with. Brain cancer patients have to consider swelling and inflammation when choosing a treatment. Too much swelling can be very dangerous since you are dealing with a limited space inside of the skull. Lung cancer patients also need to be aware that inflammation and swelling could be dangerous. There are protocols that deal with minimal to virtually no inflammation.

Lung cancer is not a type of cancer where you can comfortably combine several different therapies. A therapy that kills cancer cells too quickly can cause a substantial amount of congestion. Fortunately, for the majority of the therapies, there is typically expert phone support or even Skype for those who are unable to travel and are administering these protocols at home. They will be able to advise you further as to what you can expect.

Probably the number 1 most important issue determining the efficacy of any type of treatment, as I mentioned previously, is your state of mind. Do you want to live? Are you confident your cancer can be defeated? Are you determined to give it all that you have?

Many patients have sadly reached a perverse and absolute state of complete denial. They are so hopelessly committed mentally to the opinion and authority of their conventional doctor, the very thought or mention of alternative possibilities is totally and most assuredly, incomprehensible.

I just talked with a friend who has a close friend that has personally just given up. His conventional doctor has written him off with no further options. He has been given up and labeled a lost cause by conventional medicine. He is depressed and without any sliver of hope, he wants to die and be done with it. He is sadly and most seriously considering suicide.

I tried to explain that maybe he was depressed from the massive build-up of lactic acid and an incredibly acidic environment within his body fluids and bloodstream. That's the ash that the fire of cancer leaves behind. The friend more or less balked at the mention and absurdity of alternative therapies and the chances for any type of hope, let alone the possibility of favorable results.

One of his more than brilliant deductions was that very rich people and celebrities die all the time from cancer, surely they are rich and would know all about any chance for something alternative that might work. Does he really think that because they are rich and because they are celebrities that they are more open minded, more observant, more perceptive and in tune with the potentials of natural medicine? Is "Mensa" a part of Hollywood now? Really?.

I would think just the opposite. Since they are so wealthy and such big time Hollywood celebrities, I think they would be less likely to turn to alternative therapies. If you think about it, they can afford and are attended by the best and the brightest conventional doctors in the world. They are overly impressed and blinded by the esteemed brilliance and incredible pretentiousness of retaining the most accomplished doctors conventional medicine has to offer. Anything remotely removed from the recommendations of that noble and enlightened medical authority would be inconceivable, ludicrous and outright preposterous. Ha!

Oh well, some people are stuck in the conventional mud and the deceptive brainwashing pool of allopathic medicine. They have firmly and most unfortunately left there consciousness blinded to the wonders of God and the incredibly miraculous body He so intricately conceived.

That's ultimately what it all comes down to. It's not some amazing new and improved piece of dirt or exotic rock that cures cancer. It's brave and imaginative researchers and scientists trying to figure out how to correct and repair God's perfect design. They search for His ultimate blueprint and try and figure out how to put the torn pages of the body back together.

That's what alternative, natural medicine really is, trying to think like God. What did we take away or deposit in the body that wasn't in His original architecture? What's not supposed to be there? What number or decimal point is missing from God's original equation? Put it back, take out the trash and observe what happens. From there, the magical and magnificent beauty and synchronicity of the body has a chance to renew itself from the inside out.

You have to open your mind, expand your consciousness. Flush your denial of the impossible. What events or discoveries have come about that flustered your mind originally? Events and discoveries that seemed to be so futuristic and so incredibly mind bending and yet unbelievably, today are commonplace?

So many things categorized as pure insanity and so far fetched they seemed laughable at the time but are now a part of our evolution in reality. I bet you can think of quite a few. There's no reason why you can't be one of them too?

The battle is won or lost in your mind far before your body even has a chance. Have you lost your will to live? Is cancer your E ticket ride out of this life. Your spade in the hole. An excuse to throw in the towel and check out prematurely. I know you are tired! I know it is hard, believe me, I got to witness it firsthand, up close and personal. Who will forever be affected by your permanent absence and scarred by the fact that you didn't pursue every remote possibility?

If you or someone you know, prior to their cancer diagnosis, was fairly happy and pretty well balanced emotionally, but now, with this cancer diagnosis and challenge, a different person altogether. You need to question whether or not it is the leftover metabolic waste of cancer affecting their clarity. Is there room to push? Do you have it in you to stay connected and committed to that persons recovery and perseverance?

Many cancer patients, from conventional therapies, and from the cancer itself, become so overloaded with lactic acid their personalities change. Some change drastically. This lactic acid causes the majority of pain in cancer patients and severely suppresses and depresses the immune system, including cognitive function. This can obscure their personality and cloud their judgment.

This is when the patient needs outside intervention. They are not thinking clearly, they are not themselves. If this is the case then someone needs to recognize this and intervene! Their thought processes have been impaired by the side effects and by-products of cancer and or its treatments. They may very well want to live but are so affected by this lactic acid and other toxic build-up, their thinking and reasoning power is severely limited and declining. Don't let it go down like this if you have a reasonable chance to alter their fate.

I know some are so incredibly stubborn you would have to knock them out to administer any treatment. Some will succumb to the trough of self-pity. Someone needs to at least try and explain that they are feeling hopeless for a reason. It is all part of the evil of cancer. Amazing things happen every second of everyday. Sometimes they just need to be pushed, if you know what their buttons are and you think it might help then, push, push, push.

I don't mean to sound brash or cold hearted. It's just that cancer can be really ugly, sometimes it takes away someone's reasoning power, their logic is impaired. It can change who they used to be. I know there are those that are just too weak and beat up from a courageous fight already. I'm just saying not to be complicit if there is a chance their reasoning is a side effect of cancer shaping their ultimate decision.

The purpose of this book is to provide accurate information regarding the options available in alternative therapies. I began this book in the hopes that it would help someone save the time which many do not have if they have recently been diagnosed with a late stage disease.

As I stated earlier in the book, my wife was, out of the blue, diagnosed with stage IV lung cancer. I knew absolutely nothing about cancer. When our conventional doctor informed us that there was not much hope in treating her particular form of cancer with conventional therapies, I panicked. I was literally buried in books and the internet searching for something, anything that might offer some sort of salvation or hope.

Of course there are all the people you speak with and friends and family that mention someone they know who has a brother, who's friends mother's daughter has a friend of a friend that survived her cancer doing such and such. So I would spend massive amounts of hours trying to put together the pieces and realistic possibilities of what I could decipher from this 3rd party hearsay. Then you get wrapped up in all the warnings and misinformation and cover-ups and scandals and lies and deceit and on and on and on etc. It's becomes really confusing and overwhelming for someone still wet behind the ears with all this.

Who to trust, What to do? Where do I start? Which one should I try? Which ones are for real? Which ones make the most sense? Oh my, the twisted web we weave. I felt like I was trying to unscramble and decipher an encrypted code

I would really love to save someone from experiencing what I went through. If I can explain enough about a therapy that has had success treating a disease like cancer and try and explain a little bit of why and how it works, it would really be my blessing. I just want to offer up what is relevant and critical to any long term recovery and hopefully say it in a way that a 3rd party can understand and relate to it.

A great majority of people seeking alternative treatments have already exhausted conventional means and are desperate for some other form of hope and treatment. I am optimistic that this book will save someone many hours, days, weeks and months of research. Most of all, I pray that it offers hope. I had none in the beginning and then just scrambled bits and pieces from there.

It takes many many years of study to unravel the reality of information out there. I have so much respect for those individuals that have dedicated their lives to legitimate research and crystal clear, scientifically proven revelations of that research. The brave soldiers that stood in the whirlwind of threat from the medical establishment yet were honorably and ethically committed to any and all who beckoned the need of their services.

I certainly had the total and complete cancer experience being a full time caregiver, although, trying to deal with and successfully treat a stage IV lung cancer diagnosis with my experience was beyond daunting. I hope and pray that in some way this book removes at least a part of that daunting, overwhelmingness. I'm not even sure that is a word but you know what I'm saying, and it seems to convey my emotions, so I'm going to leave it. Sorry spell check.

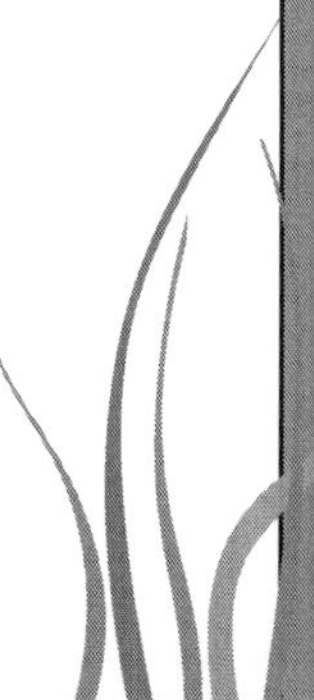

Judgment Day

The story of Alternative cancer treatments and the money and power hiding behind the oversized wallets of the current medical authority is a rough and bumpy road of deception. It rips at the core of who we are, who we have become as an evolved, refined and civilized species. It weighs out the good against the evil and breaks it down to its very nakedness. The lethal exposure that is hidden beneath the veil of corporate money mongers who would rather fill their swimming pools with the blood of innocent lives than the gold that flows from the soul and spirit of the Divine. It wreaks of an abomination of sin and darkness that simple nomenclature cannot describe. It imperils the very essence and truth of our existence, a footprint in our journey, a journey in evolution beyond the barbaric neanderthals, a journey wrought and shaped by the silver that corrodes man's mindlessness and lust for imperishable power.

In GOD we trust! I pray that you will put your Faith where it needs to be. Look up, He will never leave you.......

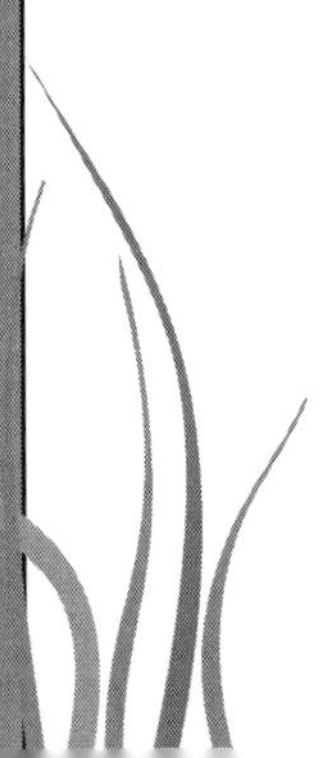

Bibliography

When Healing Becomes A Crime: The Amazing Story of The Hoxsey Cancer Clinics and The Return of Alternative Therapies...by Kenny Ausubel

Options: The Alternative Cancer Therapy Book... by Richard Walters

Outsmart Your Cancer: Alternative Non-Toxic Treatments That Work...by Tanya Harter Pierce

The Gerson Therapy: The Proven Nutritional Program for Cancer and Other Illnesses...by Charlotte Gerson & Morton Walker, D.P.M.

Healing/The Gerson Way...Second Edition/Defeating Cancer and Other Chronic Diseases... by Charlotte Gerson with Beata Bishop

The Wonders of Colloidal Silver...Natures Super Antibiotic...by Dhyana L. Coburn & Patrick D. Dignan

An Alternative Medicine Definitive Guide to Cancer...by John W. Diamond M.D. & Lee W. Cowden M.D.

The Cancer Cure That Worked! Fifty Years of Suppression...by Barry Lynes

War On Cancer: One Physician Is Winning...by Dr. Nicholas Gonzalez...Life Extension Magazine

Cancertutor.com...Webmaster and Alternative Cancer Researcher ...Webster Kehr

Flood Your Body With Oxygen...by Ed McCabe

The Miracle Of Fasting...by Paul C. Bragg N.D., Ph.D. & Patricia Bragg N.D., Ph.D.

How To Fight Cancer And Win...by William L. Fischer

Flax Oil As A True Aid Against Arthritis, Heart Infarction, Cancer and Other Diseases...Dr. Johanna Budwig

The Cure For All Cancers...by Hulda Regehr Clark Ph.D., N.D.

The Tao Of Detox...by Daniel Reid

The Cure...by Timothy Brantley Ph.D., N.D.

Cancer Cover-Up...by Kathleen Deoul

Alkalize Or Die...by Dr. Theodore A. Baroody

World Without Cancer: The Story of Vitamin B17...by G. Edward Griffin

Worldwithoutcancer.org

Nutritional Implications... by Ernest T. Krebs

Cancer: Curing the Incurable Without Surgery, Chemotherapy or Radiation...by William Donald Kelley and Fred Rohe

Cancer Therapy: The Independent Consumer's Guide to Non-Toxic Treatment and Prevention...by Ralph W. Moss, Ph.D.

Cancer—A Second Opinion...by Josef Issels, M.D.

Root Canal Cover-Up...by George E. Meinig D.D.S., F.A.C.D.

It's All In Your Head: The Link Between Mercury Amalgams and Illness...by Dr. Hal A. Huggins

You're Not Sick, Your Thirsty...by F. Batmanghelidj, M.D.

Detox For Life...by Loree Taylor Jordan, C.C.H., I.D.

Dr. Jensen's Guide To Better Bowel Care...Dr. Bernard Jensen

Made in the USA
San Bernardino, CA
07 October 2014